Primary Care for School-Aged Children

Editor

ELIZABETH K. MCCLAIN

PRIMARY CARE:
CLINICS IN OFFICE PRACTICE

www.primarycare.theclinics.com

Consulting Editor
JOEL J. HEIDELBAUGH

March 2015 • Volume 42 • Number 1

ELSEVIER

1600 John F. Kennedy Boulevard • Suite 1800 • Philadelphia, Pennsylvania, 19103-2899

http://www.theclinics.com

PRIMARY CARE: CLINICS IN OFFICE PRACTICE Volume 42, Number 1
March 2015 ISSN 0095-4543, ISBN-13: 978-0-323-35663-3

Editor: Jessica McCool
Developmental Editors: Yonah Korngold and Colleen Viola

Primary Care: Clinics in Office Practice (ISSN: 0095–4543) is published quarterly by Elsevier Inc., 360 Park Avenue South, New York, NY 10010-1710. Months of issue are March, June, September, and December. Periodicals postage paid at New York, NY and additional mailing offices. Subscription prices are $225.00 per year (US individuals), $392.00 (US institutions), $115.00 (US students), $275.00 (Canadian individuals), $444.00 (Canadian institutions), $175.00 (Canadian students), $345.00 (international individuals), $444.00 (international institutions), and $175.00 (international students). Foreign air speed delivery is included in all *Clinics* subscription prices. All prices are subject to change without notice. POSTMASTER: Send address changes to *Primary Care: Clinics in Office Practice*, Elsevier Periodicals Customer Service, 11830 Westline Industrial Drive, St. Louis, MO 63146. Customer Service Health Sciences Division, Subscription Customer Service, 3251 Riverport Lane, Maryland Heights, MO 63043. **Customer Service: 1-800-654-2452 (U.S. and Canada); 314-447-8871 (outside U.S. and Canada). Fax: 314-447-8029. E-mail: journalscustomerservice-usa@elsevier.com (for print support); journalsonlinesupport-usa@elsevier.com (for online support).**

Reprints. For copies of 100 or more, of articles in this publication, please contact the Commercial Reprints Department, Elsevier Inc., 360 Park Avenue South, New York, NY 10010-1710. Tel. 212-633-3874; Fax: 212-633-3820; E-mail: reprints@elsevier.com.

Primary Care: Clinics in Office Practice is covered in *MEDLINE/PubMed (Index Medicus) and EMBASE/ Excerpta Medica, Current Contents/Clinical Medicine, and ISI/BIOMED.*

Contributors

CONSULTING EDITOR

JOEL J. HEIDELBAUGH, MD, FAAFP, FACG
Clinical Professor, Departments of Family Medicine and Urology; Clerkship Director, Department of Family Medicine, University of Michigan Medical School, Ann Arbor, Michigan; Ypsilanti Health Center, Ypsilanti, Michigan

EDITOR

ELIZABETH K. McCLAIN, PhD, EdS, MPH
Assistant Dean, Office of Academic Affairs; Assistant Professor, Primary Care Medicine, Kansas City University of Medicine and Biosciences, College of Osteopathic Medicine, Kansas City, Missouri

AUTHORS

DEBRA AHERN, DO
Assistant Professor of Medicine, Department of Community and Family Medicine, TMC Lakewood, Kansas City, Missouri

SCOTT AKERS, DO
Resident, PGY3, Via Christi Family Medicine, Wichita, Kansas

AUBREE BRUHNDING, BS
College of Osteopathic Medicine, Kansas City University of Medicine and Biosciences, Kansas City, Missouri

ERIN JEWELL BURKS, DO
Department of Psychiatry, University of Missouri-Kansas City School of Medicine, Kansas City, Missouri

ANDREA COURTEMANCHE, PhD
Post-doctoral Fellow, Psychology, Center for Child Health and Development, University of Kansas Medical Center, Kansas City, Kansas

EMILY DIXON, DO
Faculty, Bethesda Family Practice and Sports Medicine Fellowship, Trihealth Orthopedic and Spine Institute, Cincinnati, Ohio

KATHRYN ELLERBECK, MD, FAAP
Associate Professor of Pediatrics, Center for Child Health and Development, University of Kansas Medical Center, Kansas City, Kansas

STEFANIE R. ELLISON, MD
Associate Professor, Department of Emergency Medicine, Truman Medical Center, University of Missouri-Kansas City School of Medicine, Kansas City, Missouri

JOY M. FULBRIGHT, MD
Director, Survive & Thrive Program; Assistant Professor, Division of Pediatric Hematology/Oncology/Bone Marrow Transplant, Children's Mercy Hospital, Kansas City, Missouri

LISA S. GILMER, MD, FAAP
Associate Professor, Department of Pediatrics, University of Kansas School of Medicine, Kansas City, Kansas

KEVIN F. GINN, MD
Director, Neuro-Oncology Program; Assistant Professor, Division of Pediatric Hematology/Oncology/Bone Marrow Transplant, Children's Mercy Hospital, Kansas City, Missouri

ERIN M. GUEST, MD
Assistant Professor, Division of Pediatric Hematology/Oncology/Bone Marrow Transplant, Children's Mercy Hospital, Kansas City, Missouri

MIRANDA M. HUFFMAN, MD, MEd
Assistant Professor, Department of Community and Family Medicine, University of Missouri-Kansas City, Missouri

RICHARD D. MAGIE, DO, RPh, FAAP, FACOP
Chairman, Associate Professor, Department of Pediatrics, College of Osteopathic Medicine, Kansas City University of Medicine and Biosciences, Kansas City, Missouri

CARLENE A. MAYFIELD, MPH
Research Assistant, Department of Physiology, Kansas City University of Medicine and Biosciences, Kansas City, Missouri

ELIZABETH K. McCLAIN, PhD, EdS, MPH
Assistant Dean, Office of Academic Affairs; Assistant Professor, Primary Care Medicine, Kansas City University of Medicine and Biosciences, College of Osteopathic Medicine, Kansas City, Missouri

RANCE McCLAIN, DO, FACOFP, FAOASM
Associate Professor, Osteopathic Manipulative Medicine, Kansas City University of Medicine and Biosciences, College of Osteopathic Medicine, Kansas City, Missouri

HOA NGUYEN, DO
Resident, PGY3, Via Christi Family Medicine, Wichita, Kansas

MOHAMED RADHI, MD
Associate Professor, Division of Pediatric Hematology/Oncology/Bone Marrow Transplant, Children's Mercy Hospital, Kansas City, Missouri

MITZI SCOTTEN, MD, FAAP
Associate Professor of Pediatrics; Director, Pediatric Medical Student Clerkship; Director, Pediatric Cystic Fibrosis Clinic, University of Kansas Medical Center, Kansas City, Kansas

CATHERINE SMITH, PhD
Associate Professor of Pediatrics, Center for Child Health and Development, University of Kansas Medical Center, Kansas City, Kansas

G. MARCUS STEPHENS, DO, FAAFP
Clinical Associate Professor, Kansas City University of Medicine and Biosciences; Clinical Assistant Professor, University of Kansas School of Medicine-Wichita; Osteopathic Program Director, Via Christi Family Medicine Residency, Wichita, Kansas

RICHARD R. SUMINSKI, PhD, MPH
Associate Professor, Department of Physiology, Kansas City University of Medicine and Biosciences, Kansas City, Missouri

ANNE VANGARSSE, MD, FAAP
Assistant Professor, Department of Pediatrics, College of Osteopathic Medicine, Kansas City University of Medicine and Biosciences, Kansas City, Missouri

HEIDI WOXLAND, DO
Resident, PGY3, Via Christi Family Medicine, Wichita, Kansas

Contents

of cancer when managing common childhood diseases. This article presents an overview of common pediatric cancers, their presentations, and how the primary care physician can work up patients whom they suspect have a malignancy. The goal is to help primary care doctors in early recognition and appropriate referral of patients, in order for patients to receive required specialized care in a timely manner.

Adolescent sudden cardiac death is rare. When it occurs, it is devastating to families and communities because of the unexpected nature of the death and the age of the victim. It is especially troubling because these patients are seemingly healthy compared with their adult counterparts who die from coronary artery disease. This article reviews the incidence, etiology, prevalence, risk, screening, and prevention strategies for the sudden cardiac death of adolescents.

This article discusses the relative risk of concussion/mild traumatic brain injury in school-aged children competing in athletics. It covers the initial assessment and diagnosis of concussion/mild traumatic brain injury. It also discusses the appropriate monitoring of any ongoing symptoms, and how to identify and address prolonged symptomatology. Finally, the current practice guidelines for return-to-play criteria are discussed, as well as the assessment of an athlete's risk of suffering from second impact syndrome.

Autism spectrum disorder (ASD) is both common and complicated. Many children with ASD are not identified until school age. The primary care physician (PCP) plays a vital role in recognizing the symptoms of ASD and in making referrals for definitive diagnosis. Most children with ASD also have co-occurring learning, medical, and/or mental health problems that require collaboration across the educational, medical, and mental health systems. This article reviews the symptoms of ASD, screening tools for school-aged children suspected of having ASD, and the PCP's role in identifying ASD and managing co-occurring conditions in the primary care medical home.

Attention-deficit/hyperactivity disorder (ADHD) is the most frequently diagnosed neurodevelopmental disorder; 6.4 million children and adolescents have been diagnosed with ADHD as of 2011. However, only 3.5 million children and adolescents are taking medication for ADHD. Adolescents with ADHD are much less willing to pursue or adhere to medication or psychosocial therapy, often because of their perceptions of side effects or perceived value of treatment, which places them at greater risk for difficulties at school, work, and home environments. Providing adolescents with increased autonomy through patient-centered approaches can increase their involvement and ability to manage their ADHD symptoms and treatment.

of treatment goals (weight maintenance vs weight loss) and treatment methodologies. Special emphasis needs to be made to support a child's development of healthy behavior choices. The use of medications should be avoided when possible because long-term health effects of pharmacotherapy treatment in children are unknown.

PRIMARY CARE: CLINICS IN OFFICE PRACTICE

RELATED INTEREST

Pediatric Clinics of North America, August 2014 (Vol. 61, Issue 4)
Pediatric Hospital Medicine and Pediatric Palliative Care
Mary C. Ottolini, Christina K. Ullrich, and Joanne Wolfe, *Editors*
Available at: http://www.pediatric.theclinics.com/

DOWNLOAD
Free App!

Review Articles
THE CLINICS

NOW AVAILABLE FOR YOUR iPhone and iPad

Foreword

School-Aged Children: Learn the Statistics

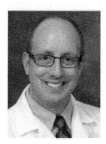

Joel J. Heidelbaugh, MD, FAAFP, FACG
Consulting Editor

I've been a family physician for over 15 years, and for the first 10 years, I practiced full-spectrum family medicine, including obstetrics. It's been amazing to see how many children I delivered now range from preschool to high school ages! Caring for some of these children reaches far beyond the standard well-child examination. While many of them are most often well, it has become quite commonplace to diagnose asthma and obesity, and I have had the unfortunate experience of diagnosing hypertension, cancer, and even life-threatening cardiac conditions. Even more unfortunate is when a child in your practice dies unexpectedly, yet the opportunity to provide comfort and support to the family and siblings makes the call of being a physician worthwhile.

In the past few decades, we've seen some mind-boggling statistics become even more unbelievable. As of Spring 2014, 1 in 68 US children had been characterized with autism spectrum disorder.[1] As of 2011, approximately 11% of children aged 4 to 17 years, or 6.4 million US children, had been diagnosed with attention deficit hyperactivity disorder (ADHD).[2] The average age of diagnosis of ADHD is 7 years, with 13.2% of boys and 5.6% of girls having the diagnosis.[2] It's hard to get through a day in my practice without seeing a child with one of these conditions. Seeing so many children with either ADHD or autism (or both) makes me ponder how many potential children go undiagnosed and struggle mightily in school, while forecasting what challenges lie ahead for them as adults in society.

One of the greatest enigmas in medicine today is the issue of food and environmental allergies. Sure, I took immunology in medical school in the 1990s, but I don't remember being impressed with the vast array of allergies we see in our children today, and the potential grave danger associated with them. Seasonal allergies always seem to be prevalent in one form or another, but I'm struggling to remember hearing of a fellow child during any of my school years who had a food allergy. Both of my daughters have severe food allergies, and safeguarding against them has been both an

http://dx.doi.org/10.1016/j.pop.2014.11.002
0095-4543/15/$ – see front matter © 2015 Published by Elsevier Inc.
primarycare.theclinics.com

education and a challenge. I also keep forgetting that EpiPens are temperature sensitive and you can't always leave them in the car!

Dr Elizabeth McClain and her colleagues have created a first-class reference that will certainly enhance the skills of family physicians, pediatricians, emergency department physicians, and allied health professionals who care for school-aged children. There are several novel topics included in this issue that merit accolades. An article dedicated to parental health literacy and its impact on the care of the school-aged child provides a solid introduction to this edition of *Primary Care: Clinics in Office Practice*. A host of articles highlighting the topics referenced above not only are current in their references and guidance but also provide practical tips for everyday practice to improve outcomes and appropriately manage pharmacotherapy. The final article addresses strategies to manage pediatric obesity, a growing epidemic that many of us often feel helpless in combatting. Augmenting our knowledge on these important topics will make us better clinicians in caring for school-aged children, and the future adults that they will become, while many of these conditions may likely linger into adulthood and present challenges for life-long health.

Joel J. Heidelbaugh, MD, FAAFP, FACG
Departments of Family Medicine and Urology
University of Michigan Medical School
Ann Arbor, MI 48109, USA

Ypsilanti Health Center
200 Arnet Suite 200
Ypsilanti, MI 48198, USA

E-mail address:
jheidel@umich.edu

REFERENCES

1. Centers for Disease Control and Prevention. CDC estimates 1 in 68 children has been identified with autism spectrum disorder. Available at: http://www.cdc.gov/media/releases/2014/p0327-autism-spectrum-disorder.html. Accessed November 22, 2014.
2. Centers for Disease Control and Prevention. Attention deficit hyperactivity disorder. Data and statistics. Available at: http://www.cdc.gov/ncbddd/adhd/data.html. Accessed November 22, 2014.

Preface

Primary Care for School-Aged Children

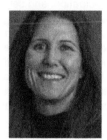

Elizabeth K. McClain, PhD, EdS, MPH
Editor

Addressing the needs of children and adolescents is a fulfilling yet challenging role for health care providers. Primary care providers play an increasingly important part delivering service through the development from childhood to young adulthood. Primary care pediatricians and adolescent health care providers are faced with daily challenges in prevention, diagnosis, and continued care. Advances in knowledge revolutionize care, through both improvements in early assessment and treatment of children and adolescents in order to improve adherence, and in the health outcomes for a broad array of health conditions. When caring for children and adolescents, physicians are challenged with mastering the art of medicine by balancing an effective yet unique relationship with the child patient, as well as developing and maintaining a supportive relationship with the adult providing care to that child. Strong communication skills and understanding of health literacy can positively impact the physician's effectiveness in delivering that care.

The first article in this issue focuses on the impact of parental health literacy on children's health. Health literacy is considered a primary factor in adherence to health behaviors and health outcomes, and individuals with lower health literacy access care when they are sicker compared to individuals with higher levels of health literacy.[1] The article provides insight as well as hands-on cases in order to foster engaged learning of how to improve health literacy with your patients.

Prevention, diagnosis, and treatment are the focus of the next articles, including HPV immunization updates and urinary tract infection. The pediatric oncology, sudden cardiac death syndrome, and concussion articles provide clear and detailed outlines for best practice in approaches to early diagnosis and referral. The focus of these articles provides clear and concise information to guide early diagnosis and treatment.

The following two articles address the changes in the DSM-V. The first of these two articles addresses how early diagnosis in children with autism is essential to improved outcomes. However, pediatricians and primary care physicians often feel inadequately

Prim Care Clin Office Pract 42 (2015) xv–xvi
http://dx.doi.org/10.1016/j.pop.2014.10.002
0095-4543/15/$ – see front matter © 2015 Published by Elsevier Inc.

trained to address issues surrounding autism. The authors provide a detailed and well laid-out structure to support the physician in serving as the medical home for the family. The second of these articles deals with attention deficit and hyperactivity disorder (ADHD). Although ADHD is often diagnosed in children, it creates a diverse set of challenges for adolescents, families, physicians, and health care providers. This article presents structures to facilitate the child's growth into young adulthood by providing supported transfer of skills to increase autonomy, active participation, and self-advocacy and to foster the physician-patient relationship.

Chronic disease management is covered in the final four articles, with topics on allergies, asthma, hypertension, and obesity. Physicians have noted an increase in pediatric and adult allergy concerns presented by patients and caregivers over the last decade. The article on allergies discusses the variation between intolerance and allergies as well as the diagnostic approaches and levels of treatment. Useful resource tables are also provided regarding the management of the environmental risks of allergy irritants.

Monitoring asthma can be challenging. The next article provides detailed clinical information for diagnosis and monitoring of asthma. The authors promote the importance of patient and family education and provide national guideline resources that are easy to integrate in patient care and education. The final two articles discuss the rise in the incidence of childhood obesity and hypertension. Because of this increased incidence, primary care physicians are faced with the challenge of effective medical management, assessment of risk, and addressing health behaviors in order to guide change.

The articles in this issue of *Primary Care: Clinics in Office Practice* address a wide variety of topics in education, prevention, diagnosis, treatment, and disease management. These articles provide guidelines for continued care and education as children progress to adolescence and young adulthood.

I am grateful for the commitment and expertise offered by each author. This issue would not have occurred without their dedication to the project. I also commend the knowledge and support provided by Yonah Korngold and Jessica McCool from Elsevier. They always offered prompt, friendly support and kept me on target. I also want to thank each author's family, who offer unconditional support, including my own family. Most importantly, I am grateful for the children and families who have entrusted us with their care as they challenge each of us to reach for continued excellence, yet remind us that we make a true difference one child, and one family, at a time.

Elizabeth K. McClain, PhD, EdS, MPH
Kansas City University of Medicine and Biosciences
College of Osteopathic Medicine
Kansas City, MO, USA

E-mail address:
emcclain@kcumb.edu

REFERENCE

1. National Center for Education Statistics. The health literacy of America's adults: results from the 2003 National Assessment of Adult Literacy. Washington, DC: US Department of Education; 2006.

Erratum

An error was made in the March 2014 issue of *Primary Care: Clinics in Office Practice* on page 95 in "Pharyngitis" by Ruth Weber. Reference 11 (McNally D, Shephard A, Field E. J Pharm Pharm Sci 2012) is used in relation to ambroxol, lidocaine and benzocaine lozenges in the last four sentences of the 'Topical treatment' section. However, Reference 11 is about a study on lidocaine lozenges and hexylresorcinol lozenges and is not about ambroxol or benzocaine lozenges.

Prim Care Clin Office Pract 42 (2015) xvii
http://dx.doi.org/10.1016/j.pop.2014.11.001
0095-4543/15/$ – see front matter © 2015 Elsevier Inc. All rights reserved.

Parental Health Literacy and Its Impact on Patient Care

Mitzi Scotten, MD

KEYWORDS

- Health literacy • Health literacy levels • Health literacy screening tools
- Pediatric health literacy • Assessing health literacy

KEY POINTS

- General health literacy is the greatest individual factor affecting a person's health status.
- Health literacy skills are grouped into the categories of clinical, preventive, and navigational ability.
- Health literacy is categorized into 4 levels: proficient, intermediate, basic, or below basic.
- Multiple health literacy tools exist that can be administered in less than 5 minutes.
- Children of parents with low literacy may have worse health outcomes.

A 12-month-old is referred to infant-toddler services to evaluate speech and motor skills that are slightly delayed on developmental testing. Despite several referrals, the family has not filled out the required paperwork for the program. At a return appointment, the clinic nurse asks the mother about the form and is handed the paperwork with many of the questions left blank. As she sits and reads the form aloud to the parent, she realizes that the mother cannot understand many of the questions and has been too embarrassed to ask for assistance.

INTRODUCTION

The process of navigating through the modern American health care system is becoming progressively more challenging. The range of tasks asked of patients in the digital age is vast and complex. These tasks can include completing intricate insurance applications, signing complex consent forms, and translating medical data and prescription medication directions. Nearly 9 out of 10 adults have difficulty using the everyday health information that is routinely offered by medical providers. Mounting evidence now supports a growing awareness that general health literacy is the greatest individual factor affecting a person's health status (**Fig. 1**).[1,2]

Pediatric Medical Student Clerkship, Pediatric Cystic Fibrosis Clinic, University of Kansas Medical Center, 3901 Rainbow Boulevard, Kansas City, KS 66160, USA
E-mail address: mscotten@kumc.edu

Prim Care Clin Office Pract 42 (2015) 1–16
http://dx.doi.org/10.1016/j.pop.2014.09.009   **primarycare.theclinics.com**

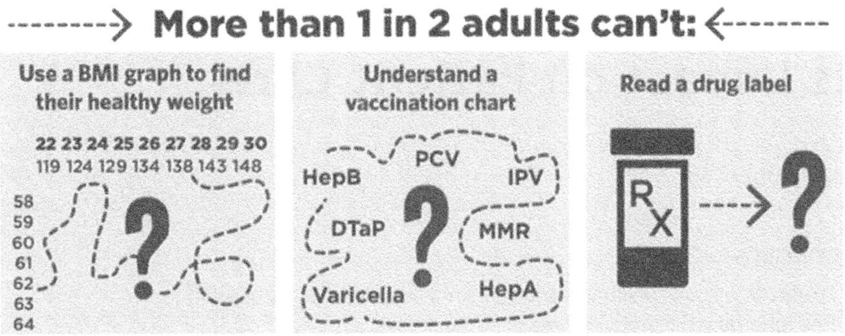

Fig. 1. General health literacy statistics. BMI, body mass index; DTaP, diphtheria tetnus acellular pertussis vaccine; HepA, hepatitis A; HepB, hepatitis B; IPV, inactivated polio vaccine; MMR, measles mumps rubella; PCV, pneumococcal conjugated vaccine; RX, medical prescription. (*From* Kutner M, Greenberg E, Jin Y, et al. The health literacy of America's adults: results from the 2003 National Assessment of Adult Literacy (NCES 2006–483). US Department of Education. Washington, DC: National Center for Education Statistics; 2006. p. 6.)

WHAT IS HEALTH LITERACY?

Health literacy is a complex entity. It is broadly defined by Healthy People 2010 as the degree to which persons have the capacity to obtain, process, and understand the basic health information and services needed to make appropriate health-related decisions.[1] Like general literacy, it depends on multiple areas, including[1]:

- Understanding the written word
- Ability to read out loud
- Calculations
- Speculation on outcomes

In pediatrics, practitioners are faced with the responsibility of addressing both the parents' and children's literacy skills. There is growing evidence that health status and access to care in children may be linked to the level of parental health literacy.[2–7] It is for this reason that the importance of understanding health literacy is being recognized as a key factor in the improvement of the overall health of the American public and as a way to decrease the widening health disparities that exist across the country.

Although the field of health literacy began in the 1990s, it was not widely studied or appreciated until the 2003 National Assessment of Adult Literacy (NAAL) report was released almost a decade ago.[2] This study of 19,000 Americans was pivotal in providing an insight into the definition, staging, and initial understanding of the current state of American health literacy. Health literacy skills are functional and involve tasks that are grouped into the categories of[2]:

- Clinical ability (case 1)
- Preventive ability (case 2)
- Navigational ability (case 3)

HEALTH LITERACY TASKS

The following cases are examples of the types of health literacy task measured by the NAAL in determining overall health literacy.[2]

Case 1 (Clinical Ability)

A 6-month-old is diagnosed with bilateral otitis media. She is prescribed amoxicillin, but returns in 3 days for continued irritability and fever. The physician examines the infant and notes that both ear canals are red and contain a viscous fluid. The mother confirms that she has been instilling the amoxicillin in the child's ears rather than by mouth because of her inability to understand the directions on the prescription.

The mother's difficulty is in performing a clinical task; one that involves medication administration. Other examples of clinical task literacy are the understanding of a disease process or treatment regimen. In pediatrics, it is the caregiver's understanding of the child's clinical condition.[2] The clinical task component encompasses the broad spectrum of health provider to patient interactions that occur on a daily basis. Clinical tasks that patients perform include:

- Making phone calls to schedule appointments
- Office visit encounters
- Receiving health instructions
- Correctly taking prescribed medications.

Health care workers have the ability to greatly influence the improvement of health care delivery in this clinical task area.

Case 2 (Preventive Ability)

A 15-year-old with insulin-dependent diabetes has been admitted to the hospital 3 times in the last 6 months for increased blood sugar levels. Although she has received education on insulin administration and diabetes management, a nurse reports that the patient was unable to calculate her insulin dose this morning for breakfast based on the carbohydrate-to-insulin calculation of 1 unit per 15 g. The patient is not checking daily blood sugar readings at home and admits to a diet high in junk food and soft drinks.

The second of the health-related tasks are preventive behaviors; in this case, the management and daily care of controlling a chronic medical condition such as type 1 diabetes. Preventive tasks involve healthy behaviors and lifestyles.[2] In pediatrics, preventive tasks are largely related to the initial years in a child's life. They include parental understanding in the importance of disease prevention methods such as breastfeeding, vaccinations, and well-child visits. As is the case in this patient with diabetes, health literacy behaviors are closely interconnected. Health preventive tasks and clinical tasks inherently depend on each other. Patients need an understanding of their specific medical conditions and also how lifestyle choices affect disease progression.

Case 3 (Navigational Ability)

A 17-year-old with cystic fibrosis is admitted to the hospital and divulges that she has not renewed her Medicaid, despite multiple conversations with the team social worker. She states that she has called several times but is put on hold for long periods of time and does not know where to go to apply in person. She is not on supplemental security income because she does not understand it and cannot find the paperwork needed to complete the application. She has not refilled medications for several months and has lost her most recent insurance card.

The last health-related task is navigational literacy and this case emphasizes the increased amount of paperwork needed to successfully receive health care in the twenty-first century. Navigation through the medical arena may include:

- Finding facilities in large medical institutions
- Keeping track of multiple appointments
- Following maps needed to locate clinics in multiple locations

It also relates to people's understanding of their rights to health care and responsibilities for payment.[2] For many, it means showing persistence and resiliency in dealing with the growing complexity that is inherent in the current medical system.

HEALTH LITERACY LEVELS

One way to assess health literacy is to categorize a person into 1 of 4 levels:

- Proficient
- Intermediate
- Basic
- Below basic

Fig. 2 and **Table 1** provide overviews of American literacy rates and abilities associated with each level.

A proficient level allows people to perform complex health care tasks that may be needed for comparisons and calculations of critical risk-benefit decisions. These skills are routine in completing standard medical paperwork such as power of attorney or insurance forms. They are also required in making high-stakes decisions based on odds ratios, such as choosing the therapy options needed for cancer treatment. It is estimated that only 12% of Americans function in this range.[2]

At the intermediate proficiency level, a patient can perform moderately challenging tasks such as:

- Reviewing a chart to identify when a child will need a vaccination
- Reading food labels to identify grams of fat per serving
- Making inferences from medical literature
- Understanding cause and effect of a particular treatment or medication regimen

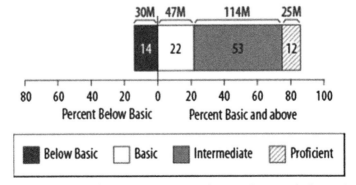

Fig. 2. Health literacy levels. (*From* Kutner M, Greenberg E, Ying J, et al. Literacy in everyday life: results from the 2003 National Assessment of Adult Literacy. US Department of Education; 2007.)

Health Literacy Level	Score Range	Task Competency
Table 1 **American health literacy scoring system**		
Below basic	0–184	Can identify a concrete activity to perform on simple, brief set of instructions
		Can read instructions using words with few syllables and in simple short sentences
		Graphics are useful for emphasis and illustration
Basic	185–225	Can read narrative using simple words and declarative statements
		Can extract major points of information from narrative with middle-school readability level
		Graphics are useful for emphasis and illustration
Intermediate	226–309	Can accurately read prescription labels and take the medicine according to directions
		Can apply information to the use of a scale to locate answer; eg, growth charts, development charts
		Can interpret information presented in narrative or graphic format
Proficient	310–500	Able to compare and contrast different sources of information
		Understands difficult abstract concepts pertaining to medical information
		Able to calculate share of costs pertaining to health insurance plan of coverage

(*Adapted from* Kutner M, Greenberg E, Ying J, et al. Literacy in everyday life: results from the 2003 National Assessment of Adult Literacy. US Department of Education; 2007.)

It is thought that most Americans (about 53%) function in an intermediate capacity.[2] Patients in the intermediate level can still find certain aspects of health care confusing. They may also make poor health care decisions because of an inadequate understanding of the many nuances related to the system.

People in the basic literacy range can:

- Review a simple pamphlet
- Understand why they are being tested for a disease for which they show no symptoms
- Calculate what times they should take a medication using 2 pieces of information
- Fill in birth dates and names on a health insurance form

Twenty-two percent of Americans are thought to function at a basic level.[2] The risk for those with basic literacy may be as serious as those with below basic literacy because of the potential inability of providers to identify this group. Those with basic skills may seem to be functioning at a higher literacy level.[2]

For those with below basic health literacy, estimated at 14%, medical information is understood only when presented in very basic prose and tables.[2] The NAAL recommends that information to this group:

- Be at the third grade reading level
- Contain mathematical tasks that involve addition only
- Be provided via short, concrete forms
- Should have the important facts circled or highlighted

Examples of below basic literacy include finding information on what time parents need to stop feeding their child before a procedure or signing a form for vaccinations. For pediatricians, this means that parents of below basic level are unlikely to comprehend:

- Over-the-counter medication dosing information
- When a child should receive a vaccination based on a printed schedule table
- A standard body mass index (BMI) graph to understand their child's weight

Parents with below basic health literacy are more likely to have not completed a high school education, to speak a language other than English before entering school, and to have no health insurance.[2] The acquisition of health-related information is more likely to be obtained via television or radio in the below basic group and from the Internet in the proficient group. Access to the Internet is increasing for the general population, but it is estimated that most health-related sites are written at the ninth grade level or greater (**Fig. 3**).[2]

Health Literacy Measurement Tools

Tests designed to measure health literacy are not widely known or used by most clinicians in current practice. Although opinion in the late 1990s was that measurement of health literacy in the office was too cumbersome, there are new resources to potentially change those views.

Initial literacy assessments, such as the Test of Functional Health Literacy in Adults (TOFHLA), were too long to administer in the nonresearch setting and required education on administration and scoring. With increased awareness of the need for literacy measurement, several well-studied and validated tools now have shorter versions and new tools have emerged to fill the need for faster assessment. Health care professionals have a growing assortment of validated tools to use for the measurement of health literacy in parents, and a lesser number available for use in children.[3,8–10]

Percentage of adults who got information about health issues
from TV (left) vs. Internet (right), by health literacy level.

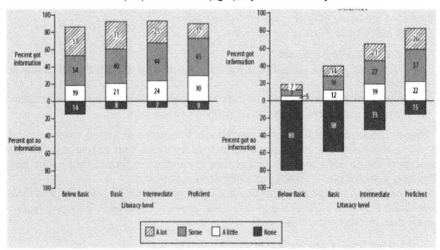

Fig. 3. Health literacy information sources. (*From* Kutner M, Greenberg E, Ying J, et al. Literacy in everyday life: the health literacy of America's adults: results from the 2003 National Assessment of Adult Literacy. US Department of Education; 2006.)

Current quick tools to measure health literacy include:

- Rapid Assessment of Adult Literacy in Medicine–Short Form (REALM-SF)
- S-TOFHLA
- Newest Vital Sign (NVS)

All three have the capability of being administered in less than 5 minutes. Pediatricians can access the tests online and download specific instructions for delivery and scoring. Test results are easy to understand and usually divide individuals into 3 or 4 categories of literacy. The NVS tool (**Fig. 4**) can be delivered to children as young as 7 years of age.[3]

A cross-sectional study by Sanders and colleagues[4] in 2004 found that the screening question of "How many children's books do you have in the home?" had a high correlation with parental literacy. Families with more than 10 children's books in the home had a 91% positive predictive value for adequate literacy.

With few tools currently available to quickly measure children's literacy levels, it is important for pediatricians to monitor for low literacy at annual visits. Examples include:

- Asking parents about grade level reading skills
- Asking children for their views on reading (**Box 1**, **Fig. 5**)
- Providing assistance with schools to develop individualized learning plans
- Encouraging parents to read aloud to children
- Using programs such as Reach Out and Read to provide books to children at well-child visits

Pediatric Outcomes and Health Literacy

The area of health literacy and pediatrics has not been studied extensively. A systematic review of the literature in 2009 found only 24 pediatric articles meeting inclusion

READ TO SUBJECT: This information is on the back of a container of a pint of ice cream.

QUESTIONS

1. If you eat the entire container, how many calories will you eat?
   Answer 1,000 is the only correct answer

2. If you are allowed to eat 60 g of carbohydrates as a snack, how much ice cream could you have?
   Answer Any of the following is correct:
   1 cup (or any amount up to 1 cup
   Half the container
   Note: If patient answers, "2 servings", ask "How much ice cream would that be if you were to measure it into a bowl?"

3. Your doctor advises you to reduce the amount of saturated fat in your diet. You usually have 42 g of saturated fat each day, which includes 1 serving of ice cream. If you stop eating ice cream, how many grams of saturated fat would you be consuming each day?
   Answer 33 is the only correct answer

4. If you usually eat 2,500 calories in a day, what percentage of your daily value of calories will you be eating if you eat one serving?
   Answer 10% is the only correct answer

Pretend you are allergic to the following substances: Penicillin, peanuts, latex gloves, and bee stings:

5. Is it safe for you to eat this ice cream?
   Answer No

6. (Ask only if the patient responds "no" to question) Why not?
   Answer Because it has peanut oil.

ANSWER CORRECT?	
YES	NO
___	___
___	___
___	___
___	___
___	___
___	___
Total Correct	___

Nutrition Facts

Serving Size	½ cup
Servings per container	4

Amount per serving

Calories 250	Fat Cal 120

	%DV
Total Fat 13g	20%
Sat Fat 9g	40%
Cholesterol 28mg	12%
Sodium 55mg	2%
Total Carbohydrate 30g	12%
Dietary Fiber 2g	
Sugars 23g	
Protein 4g	8%

•Percent Daily Values (DV) are based on a 2,000 calorie diet. Your daily values may be higher or lower depending on your calorie needs.

Ingredients: Cream, Skim Milk, Liquid Sugar, Water, Egg Yolks, Brown Sugar, Milkfat, Peanut Oil, Sugar, Butter, Salt, Carrageenan, Vanilla Extract.

Fig. 4. NVS screening tool example. (*From* Pfizer, Inc. The Newest Vital Sign. Available at: http://www.pfizer.com/files/health/nvs_flipbook_english_final.pdf. Copyright © Pfizer Inc. All rights reserved; used with permission.)

Box 1
Steps to enhance patient understanding

1. Slow down.

   Communication can be improved by speaking slowly, and by spending a small amount of additional time with each patient. This approach helps to foster a patient-centered approach to the clinician-patient interaction.

2. Use plain, nonmedical language.

   Explain things to patients the way you would explain them to your grandmother.

3. Show or draw pictures.

   Visual images can improve patients' recall of ideas.

4. Limit the amount of information provided, and repeat it.

   Information is best remembered when it is given in small pieces that are pertinent to the tasks at hand. Repetition further enhances recall.

5. Use the teach-back technique.

   Confirm that patients understand by asking them to repeat back your instructions.

6. Be respectful, caring, and sensitive. Encourage questions.

   Make patients feel comfortable asking questions. Enlist the aid of others (patient's family or friends) to promote understanding.

Adapted from Shuman J. Primary issues. Inadequate health literacy: a barrier to patient care. Available at: http://www.primaryissues.org/2010/04/inadequate-health-literacy-a-barrier-to-patient-care/. Accessed September 19, 2014.

---

criteria.[5] Two key questions to assess in the complex relationship of parental literacy and child outcomes are:

- What effect does low literacy level in a caregiver or child have on pediatric health and development?
- What interventions can be provided to children and caregivers with low health literacy to decrease outcome disparities?

Initial implications of low caregiver literacy are emerging and show that children of parents with low literacy skills have worse health outcomes.

Among the current associations of lower parental health literacy and pediatric outcomes are the following[5]:

- Increased emergency room visits and higher hospitalization rates in children with asthma
- Decreased parental comprehension of information included in vaccine and newborn screening brochures
- Decreased parental understanding that liquid medication is dosed on weight
- Decreased rates of breastfeeding
- Increased rates of parental smoking

Studies assessing literacy in adolescents support the continued trend in poorer health care choices with teens with lower literacy being more likely to[5]:

- Carry guns
- Smoke tobacco
- Get into fights

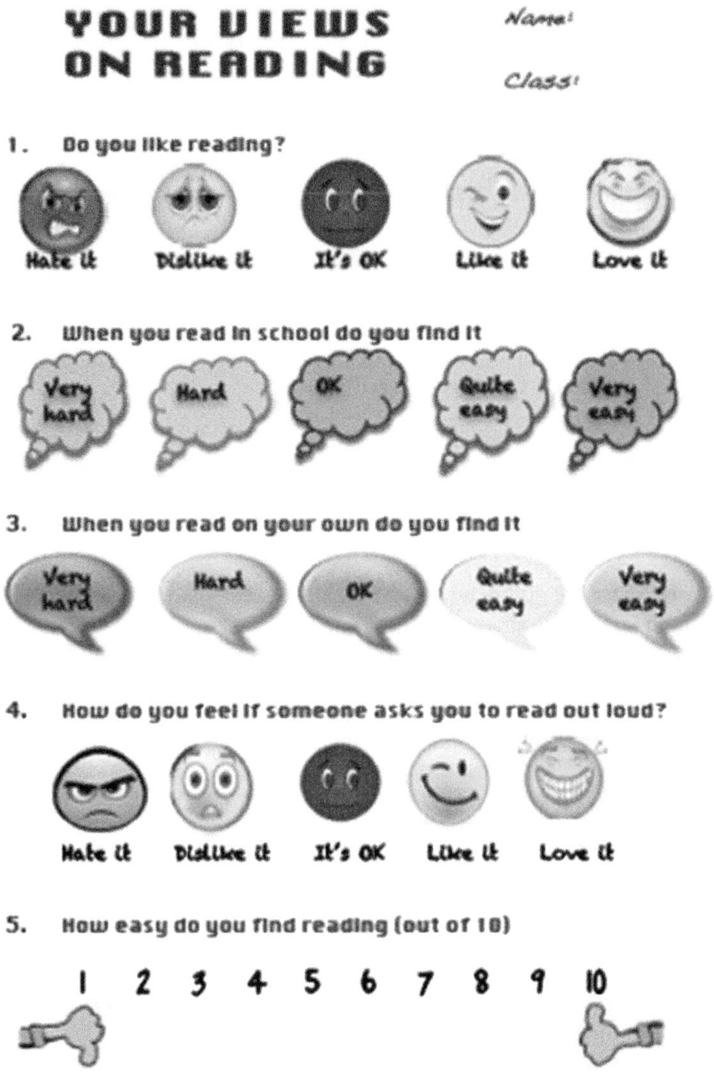

YOUR VIEWS ON READING

Name:

Class:

1. Do you like reading?

Hate it   Dislike it   It's OK   Like it   Love it

2. When you read in school do you find it

Very hard   Hard   OK   Quite easy   Very easy

3. When you read on your own do you find it

Very hard   Hard   OK   Quite easy   Very easy

4. How do you feel if someone asks you to read out loud?

Hate it   Dislike it   It's OK   Like it   Love it

5. How easy do you find reading (out of 10)

1 2 3 4 5 6 7 8 9 10

Fig. 5. Sample tool for measuring a child's view on reading. (*From* The National Behavior Support Service (NBSS). Catch Up Literacy. Available at: http://www.nbss.ie/interventions-projects/academic-literacy-and-learning/catch-up-literacy. Accessed September 19, 2014.)

Studies relating to breastfeeding and newborn screening found that a major reason for decreased parental comprehension is related to the complexity of current medical brochures and handouts given to parents.[5] For newborn screening, national and state disseminated information to parents is written at an average tenth grade reading level and primary care physicians were found to use complex medical jargon when providing genetic counseling to parents.[5] A study on breastfeeding found that more than 7 out of 10 mothers did not accurately understand information about breastfeeding after reading a page from a guide written by the American Academy of Pediatrics.[5]

Few studies have examined potential interventions in pediatric practice to improve outcomes in parents and children with low literacy and research is needed in this area. The findings of studies with interventions for low literacy include the following[5]:

- Modifying the readability of medically related documents improved comprehension in caregivers
- Using a 2-hour program and weekly camp to provide additional information and medical instruction on asthma education decreased visits to the emergency department by 30%
- The use of pictogram-based instructions and teach-back counseling resulted in significantly fewer errors in medication preparation and dosing compared with standard practice

PEDIATRICIANS' PERSPECTIVES ON HEALTH LITERACY

As primary carers at the forefront of health promotion, how do pediatricians view themselves in the area of health literacy? A national survey of more than 800 pediatricians, published in 2009, reported that most of them typically use communication techniques with patients and families to address literacy issues.[6] These techniques included:

- Use of common language when discussing medical jargon
- Repeating key information
- Detailing amounts of medication to be administered when giving prescriptions

Also reported at slightly lower rates were:

- Encouraging parents to call back for any questions
- Confirming that treatment plans were followed at subsequent visits
- Presenting only 2 to 3 concepts at a time
- Talking slowly

Seven of 10 doctors surveyed reported that they use one of these methods most of the time with patients and families.[6]

The use of more detailed and enhanced communication strategies was less common. Fifty percent or less of pediatricians reported that they:

- Wrote out specific treatment plans for parents
- Reinforced key elements of the visit
- Gave dates and times when prescribing medications
- Demonstrated how to administer medications
- Underlined key information on take-home material
- Asked parents to teach back what they had learned
- Called parents after the visit to follow up on the treatment plan

In addition, although it is the more time consuming and detailed information that seems to improve communication transfer to those with lower literacy, only a minority of providers regularly used enhanced techniques.[6]

Case 4

A 15-month-old is brought to the emergency department for lethargy and jaundice. Liver enzyme levels are increased. The parents reveal that they have been giving the patient 2 medications over the last week for cough and fever. They were advised at their last well-child visit to give children's Tylenol for fever but have been administering an additional cough and cold medicine that contains acetaminophen. The parents are not aware that they have been giving double the dosage of acetaminophen, that Tylenol and acetaminophen are the same, or that the dosing chart on the cold medication recommends discussing its use with a physician before administration.

Medication errors in the national survey reported[6] that:

- Eighty-one percent of pediatricians could recall at least 1 situation in the previous year in which parents did not understand the medical information that had been delivered
- Forty-four percent of the physicians were aware of an error in medical treatment of a child caused by parental difficulty with reading or writing skills
- The 300 physicians who described a medical error to a child in their practice stated that 15% were in the category of causing moderate to great harm

Pediatricians reported a lack of time as their most significant barrier to using enhanced communication techniques in their daily practice.[6] Other barriers cited were the increased complexity of medical information needing to be related to families and the volume of information that is required for both sick visits and well-child checks.[6] Pediatricians become adept at multitasking the delivery of information in short exchanges to children and families. However, caregivers may find it hard to fully absorb medical information and may ask for clarification on details while tending to a hungry infant, crying toddler, or overactive sibling.[7]

PRACTICE APPLICATIONS FOR PEDIATRICIANS

Starting a health literacy project in the pediatric office setting is now possible with the availability of free and easily accessible programs. One example is the Health Literacy Universal Precautions Toolkit sponsored by the Agency for Healthcare Research and Quality.[11]

Offices can use the Quick Start Guide to introduce increased health literacy awareness in 3 steps:

- The first step is to provide all employees with a brief introduction to health literacy[11]

The dissemination of health literacy awareness to the entire staff cannot be understated, given that, at any office visit, the family interacts with multiple members of the health care team.

- The second Quick Start action is to ask each provider in the practice to identify an area of communication on which to focus in their daily patient interactions and to use a recommended health literacy tool.[11]

One example is improving the understanding of instructions provided to a family in an office encounter, because it is estimated that patients forget up to 80% of what is discussed in a single visit.[11] A strategy to overcome this loss of information is the teach-back method. The teach-back method asks the patient or caregiver to demonstrate the use of equipment, such as an inhaler, back to the provider. This technique has been shown to increase the chances of successful follow-through days to weeks later, especially for patients with limited literacy.[11]

- The third action is to perform frequent assessments of the new health literacy implementations.[11]

Providers try a technique on several patients and then report to others in the group. Quality improvement measures such as the Plan-Do-Study-Act model (PDSA cycle) recommend frequent reassessment of new practices to ensure that they are working and to increase the probability of long-term sustainability and success. Health literacy policies may qualify as quality improvement requirements for physician maintenance of certification and best practice initiatives (**Fig. 6**).

SUSTAINING A HEALTH LITERACY PROGRAM

Once a health literacy program is introduced, it is important to understand that a new set of guidelines is designed ultimately to improve the health outcomes for patients. Promoting health literacy should focus on 4 key areas of operation[7,11]:

- Improved oral communication
- Improved written communication
- Improved empowerment and self-management for patients
- Improved support systems

Improved oral communication involves:

- Training all office staff in effective communication techniques
- Using enhanced communication techniques with patients
- Frequently assessing for the use of jargon when explaining the need for medical care, such as immunizations

Although 99% of pediatricians in the 2009 pediatrics survey reported using common language to their patients in everyday encounters, evidence provided by direct observation of physicians has found that more than 80% use at least 1 unclarified jargon term per medical visit.[6,7]

Written communication improvements begin with the assessment of all forms and brochures given to patients and families. Providing low-literacy options might involve[7]:

- Having paperwork with less print and tables
- The use of pictograms to explain procedures
- Having nonprint versions of important medical information
- Demonstration videos in waiting rooms to relay preventive health issues

The next step is to improve the self-management skills of children and caregivers and to empower all patients to improve their overall health.[11] Lower literacy increases

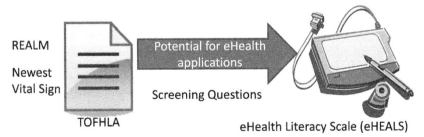

Fig. 6. Validated health literacy screening instruments. (*From* Collins SA, Curried LM, Bakken S, et al. Health literacy screening instruments for eHealth applications: a systematic review. J Biomed Inform 2012;45(3):598; with permission.)

the likelihood of poor adherence to medical regimens and is directly related to poorer control of chronic conditions.[7] Persons with low literacy are less likely to advocate for themselves or their children and, as a result, have decreased power in shared medical decision making.[11,12]

Offices can increase patient and caregiver empowerment in several ways[11]:

- Increase awareness that persons with lower literacy are less likely to ask questions during a routine medical visit
- Create an environment in the office in which questions are expected
- Provide support staff with information on how to elicit questions

In the Ask Me 3 program, through the National Patient Safety Foundation, patients are directed to increase involvement in their care by knowing the following at the end of every encounter[11]:

- What is my child's main problem?
- What do I need to know (to take care of my child)?
- Why is it important for my child to do this?

Another pertinent tool to increase self-management skills is the use of a medical action plan. Patients with lower literacy may feel less involved in a shared decision-making model and, despite recurrent medical encounters, may continue to make

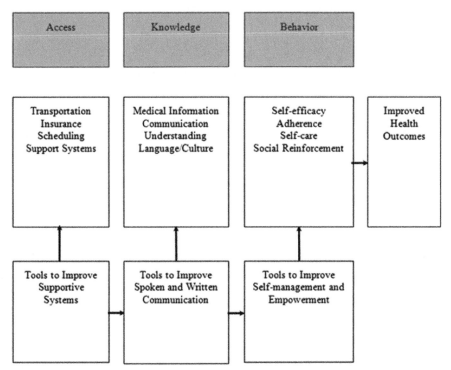

Fig. 7. Factors necessary to improve health outcomes and tools to help. (*From* US Department of Health and Human Services. Indian Health Service. Health Literacy Universal Precautions Toolkit. Available at: http://www.ihs.gov/healthcommunications/index.cfm?module5dsp_hc_health_literacy. Accessed September 19, 2014.)

poor decisions regarding their child's health.[11] Important aspects of the medical action plan are:

- Incorporating the child and family as active players
- Use of the patient's and family's own motivation and suggestions for change
- Creation of simple and realistic goals that are attainable
- Writing down the steps that are chosen for the family to take home
- Asking the family if they think that the plan is reasonable and something they can achieve before the next visit

A national trend of increased childhood obesity is an example of an area in which a pediatrician could use an action plan to work with a patient and family.

The last important step for primary care offices is to acknowledge that families with limited literacy are likely to face challenges outside the health care arena.[11] Transportation, housing, and access to affordable medications can be daunting for those with low literacy. Dealing with these challenges might include:

- Providing families with a list of community resources for assistance
- Dedicating office staff to deal primarily with families needing additional services
- Creating an environment of mutual respect and understanding for people facing limited literacy

Implementation of programs for patients with low literacy can improve the patients' chances of following through on medical tasks and can assist in the navigation of systems outside the immediate pediatric practice (**Fig. 7**).

SUMMARY

Advocates for health literacy have recommended that it be treated in the same way as blood-borne illnesses; that is, with universal precautions.[11] By designating it as a universal precaution, health literacy would be assessed in all patients, and this has the potential to decrease the chances of missing it in anyone. Other clinicians suggest that it be considered as the fifth vital sign because it is considered one of the single best predictors of a patient's general health (**Fig. 8**).[3]

Use of universal health literacy precautions makes sense because:

- The routine testing of all children and adults for literacy level is daunting and generally beyond the scope of any single pediatric practice
- Adopting the idea that problems with health literacy can, and likely do, exist for almost all Americans minimizes the delivery of care that is not understood
- Universal precautions increase the likelihood that health care consumers will have the opportunity make truly informed decisions for themselves and their children

Identification of patients with lower literacy is challenging. The silent epidemic of impaired health literacy is related to a myriad of issues but is most likely underdiagnosed for the following reasons[11]:

- Persons of limited literacy may have completed high school or even have college degrees
- They hold white collar jobs as well as blue collar jobs
- They may appear well spoken and state that they understand what they are being told
- They may look at health information given to them and say they understand it

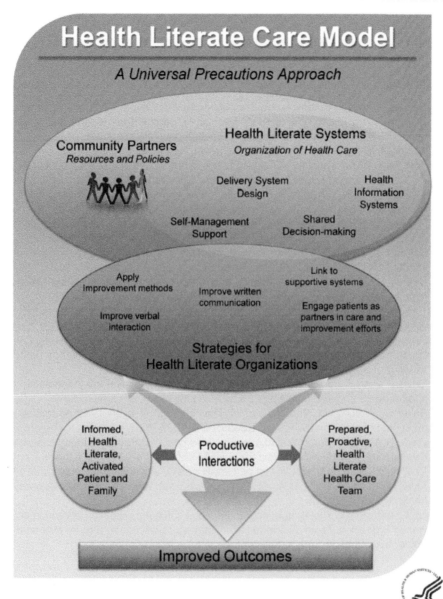

Fig. 8. Health literacy care model, showing the link between community partners, health literate systems, and health literate organizations as they interact productively with each other to improve outcomes. Community partners include resources and policies. Health literate systems focus on the organization of health care (eg, design of the delivery system, self-management support, shared decision making, and health information systems). Health literate organizations strategically apply improvement methods, improve written communication, link to supportive systems, improve verbal interaction, and engage patients as partners in care and improvement efforts. The productive interactions enable (1) families and patients to be informed, health literate, and active in care and improvement efforts; and (2) the health care team to be prepared, proactive, and health literate. (*From* Agency for Healthcare Research & Quality (AHRQ). Health literate care model. Available at: http://www.health.gov/communication/interactiveHLCM/index.html.)

- They are just as likely to be patients you think you know well as patients you have just met

REFERENCES

1. Office of Disease Prevention and Promotion. Healthy People 2010: understanding and improving health. Washington, DC: US Department of Health and Human Services; 2010. Available at: http://www.health.gov/healthypeople.
2. Kutner M, Greenberg E, Jin Y, et al. The health literacy of America's adults: results from the 2003 National Assessment of Adult Literacy (NCES 2006–483). US Department of Education. Washington, DC: National Center for Education Statistics; 2006. Available at: http://nces.ed.gov/pubsearch/pubsinfo.asp?pubid=2006483.
3. Driessnack M, Chung MA, Perkhounkova E, et al. Using the "Newest Vital Sign" to assess health literacy in children. J Pediatr Health Care 2013;28(2):165–71.
4. Sanders L, Zacur G, Haecker T, et al. Number of children's books in home: an indicator of parent health literacy. Ambul Pediatr 2004;4(5):424–8.
5. DeWalt DA, Hink A. Health literacy and child health outcomes: a systematic review of the literature. Pediatrics 2009;124(Suppl 3):S265–74.
6. Turner T, Cull W, Bayldon B, et al. Pediatricians and health literacy: descriptive results from a national survey. Pediatrics 2009;124(Suppl 3):S299–305.
7. Saunders L, Shaw J, Guez G, et al. Health literacy and child health promotion: implications for research, clinical care and public policy. Pediatrics 2009; 124(Suppl 3):S306–13.
8. Davis T, Long S, Jackson R, et al. Rapid estimate of adult literacy in medicine: a shortened instrument. Fam Med 1993;25:391–5.
9. Baker D, Williams M, Parker R, et al. Development of a brief test to measure functional health literacy. Patient Educ Couns 1999;38:33–42.
10. Weiss B, Mays M, Martz W, et al. Quick assessment of literacy in primary care: the newest vital sign. Ann Fam Med 2005;3:514–22.
11. DeWalt D, Callahan L, Hawk V, et al. Health literacy universal precautions tool kit. AHRQ Publication No.10-0046-EF. 2010. Available at: www.ahrq.gov/qual/literacy/healthliteracytoolkit.pdf.
12. US Department of Health and Human Services, Office of Disease Prevention and Health Promotion. Quick Guide to HealthLiteracy. Available at: http://www.health.gov/communication/literacy/quickguide/.

Human Papillomavirus Vaccine Update

Lisa S. Gilmer, MD

KEYWORDS

- Human papillomavirus • Human papillomavirus vaccine • Adolescent vaccination
- Cervical cancer • Genital warts

KEY POINTS

- Seventy-nine million people in the United States are currently infected with human papillomavirus (HPV).
- Fourteen million new HPV infections and 26,000 cancers attributable to HPV are diagnosed yearly.
- Every year in the United States, ~15,000 HPV-associated cancers in women and ~7000 HPV-associated cancers in men may be prevented by HPV vaccines.
- Human papillomavirus vaccine has been shown to be safe and effective.
- In 2012, only 33% of girls aged 13 to 17 years had received the 3 recommended doses of HPV vaccine.
- Health care providers play a key role in improving HPV vaccination rates.

INTRODUCTION TO HUMAN PAPILLOMAVIRUS

Genital human papillomavirus (HPV) is the most commonly diagnosed sexually transmitted infection in the United States. It is estimated that nearly all sexually active men and women have HPV at some point in their lives (**Box 1**).

Human Papillomavirus Transmission and Risk Factors

The most consistently listed HPV infection predictors are measures of sexual activity and, in particular, the number of sex partners and the number of their sex partners, and earlier age at time of first sexual encounter. Most commonly transmitted by

Funding sources: None.
Conflict of interest: None.
Department of Pediatrics, University of Kansas School of Medicine, 3901 Rainbow Boulevard, Mail Stop 4004, Kansas City, KS 66160, USA
E-mail address: lgilmer@kumc.edu

Box 1
HPV overview

- Seventy-nine million Americans are infected with HPV, with about 14 million new infections per year[1]
- Approximately 50% of the HPV infections occur in young adults aged 15 to 24 years, who represent only 25% of the sexually experienced population[2]
- Twenty-five percent of girls and women aged 14 to 19 years are infected with HPV[3]
- Every year 26,000 new cancers are attributable to HPV, including 18,000 in women and 8000 in men[4]
- Cervical cancer is the most common HPV-associated cancer among women, and oropharyngeal cancers are the most common among men
- More than 360,000 cases of genital warts occur yearly in the United States among sexually active men and women[1]

---

direct genital contact during vaginal and anal sex, it is less common for HPV to be transmitted by oral sex, genital-to-genital contact without intercourse, or from mother to newborn.[5]

Clinical Course of Human Papillomavirus Infections

Greater than 90% of HPV infections are transient and asymptomatic so adolescents may not even be aware they are infected. Most HPV infections clear within 1 to 2 years causing no sequelae. However, 10% of infections persist with the potential to cause a variety of serious health problems.[5]

HEALTH PROBLEMS CAUSED BY HUMAN PAPILLOMAVIRUS

The scope of the HPV problem in the United States is presented in **Box 2**. HPV infection can cause a variety of health problems, as shown in **Box 3**. There is no definitive way to predict which adolescents infected with HPV will go on to develop warts, cancer, or other health problems. However, the problem that may develop is determined largely by the HPV type that they contract, as listed in **Table 1**.

Box 2
Scope of HPV problem in the United States in 2013

- Genital warts: 360,000 cases
- Cervical cancer: ~12,340 new cases and 4030 deaths
- Other genital cancers: 7500 cases
- Oropharyngeal cancers: 8400 cases

Data from CDC. Recommendations on the use of quadrivalent human papillomavirus vaccine in males – Advisory Committee on Immunization Practices. MMWR Morb Mortal Wkly Rep 2011;60(50):1705–8; and National Cancer Institute. Cervical cancer. Available at: http://www.cancer.gov/cancertopics/types/cervical. Accessed February 24, 2014.

Box 3
Health problems caused by HPV

- All cases caused by HPV infection:
  - Condyloma acuminate (genital warts)
  - Recurrent respiratory papillomatosis
- Most cases caused by HPV infection:
  - Cervical cancer and cervical cancer precursors, 95% linked to HPV
- Other cancers and cancer precursors linked to HPV infection:
  - Vulvar cancers, 50% linked to HPV
  - Vaginal cancers, 65% linked to HPV
  - Penile cancers, 35% linked to HPV
  - Anal cancers, 95% linked to HPV
  - Oropharyngeal cancer, 60% linked to HPV

Adapted from CDC. Human papillomavirus-associated cancers – United States, 2004-2008. MMWR Morb Mortal Wkly Rep 2012;61(15):258–61. Available at: http://www.cdc.gov/mmwr/preview/mmwrhtml/mm6115a2.htm. Accessed February 24, 2014.

Human Papillomavirus–related Cancers

HPV is associated with several cancers in both men and women. **Table 2** summarizes data from the 2004 to 2008 National Program of Cancer Registries (NPCR) and the Surveillance, Epidemiology, and End Results (SEER) program's breakdown of HPV-associated cancers.

These numbers translate to about 1 cancer, mostly cervical, for every 175 girls born each year and 1 cancer, mostly of the head and neck, for every 300 boys born each year.[6]

Strategies for Reducing Risk of Human Papillomavirus Infection

Strategies to reduce the burden of HPV infection and related health problems should be incorporated into the routine health maintenance of adolescent patients. The following are recommendations for reducing the risk of contracting HPV infection or of developing HPV-related diseases.

Table 1
HPV subtypes and risk of future health problems

Low-risk Subtypes	High-risk Subtypes
HPV 6 and 11 cause ~90% of genital warts	HPV16 and HPV18 cause ~70% of cervical cancers
HPV 6 and 11 cause most cases of recurrent respiratory papillomatosis	In women, HPV16 is associated with cancers of the vulva, vagina, anus, and oropharynx
HPV 6 and 11 can cause benign or low-grade cervical cancers	In men, HPV16 is associated with cancers of the penis, anus, and oropharynx

Data from CDC. Quadrivalent human papillomavirus vaccine, recommendations of the Advisory Committee on Immunizations Practices. MMWR Morb Mortal Wkly Rep 2007;56(RR02):1–24. Available at: http://www.cdc.gov/mmwr/preview/mmwrhtml/rr5602a1.htm. Accessed February 24, 2014.

Table 2 HPV-associated cancers by site			
	Average Annual Number of Diagnoses	Number Attributable to HPV	Rate per 100,000 Population
Cervical	11,967	11,500	7.7
Vulvar	3136	1600	1.8
Vaginal	729	500	0.4
Penile	1046	400	0.8
Anal			
Female	3089	2900	1.8
Male	1678	1600	1.2
Oropharyngeal			
Female	2370	1500	1.4
Male	9356	5900	6.2

Data from CDC. Human papillomavirus-associated cancers – United States, 2004-2008. MMWR Morb Mortal Wkly Rep 2012;61(15):258–61. Available at: http://www.cdc.gov/mmwr/preview/mmwrhtml/mm6115a2.htm. Accessed February 24, 2014.

- Abstinence from sexual contact
- Routine condom use with every sex act
- Limiting the number of sexual partners
- For cervical cancer: cervical cancer screening for women aged 21 to 65 years
- For oropharyngeal cancers: avoidance of tobacco and limiting of alcohol consumption
- HPV vaccination

Note that the HPV vaccine does not replace the need for cervical cancer screening. The HPV vaccine in adolescents and cervical cancer screening in women should be done in tandem to reduce the incidence of cervical cancer.[7]

Summary of Health Problems Caused by Human Papillomavirus

HPV is the most commonly diagnosed sexually transmitted disease in the United States, and is the leading cause of cervical cancer, as well as a significant contributor to other urogenital cancers and oropharyngeal cancers and a cause of genital warts. There is no treatment of HPV infection, making infection prevention the best way to prevent HPV-related diseases.

HUMAN PAPILLOMAVIRUS VACCINES: HISTORY, EFFICACY, AND IMMUNOGENICITY

The first HPV vaccine was licensed for use in the United States in June 2006. At present there are 2 HPV vaccines available in the United States.

HPV4, or Human Papillomavirus Quadrivalent (Types 6, 11, 16, 18) Vaccine, Recombinant (Gardasil), is manufactured by Merck & Co, Inc. HPV4 is directed against oncogenic HPV types (16 and 18) and nononcogenic HPV types (6 and 11).[8]

HPV2, or Human Papillomavirus Bivalent (Types 16 and 18) Vaccine, Recombinant (Cervarix), is manufactured by GlaxoSmithKline Biologicals. HPV2 is directed against oncogenic HPV types (16 and 18).[9]

Human Papillomavirus Vaccine History

Fig. 1 provides a timeline for the licensure of the HPV vaccines by the US Food and Drug Administration (FDA) and the recommendations for the use of HPV vaccines by the Centers for Disease Control and Prevention (CDC) Advisory Committee for Immunization Practices (ACIP).[5,10,11]

Efficacy of Human Papillomavirus Vaccines

Both vaccines have been shown be highly efficacious. Data from clinical trials performed before licensure of HPV4 and HPV2 showed good vaccine efficacy[8]:

- Both vaccines have greater than 95% efficacy in preventing HPV16-related and HPV18-related cervical precancer lesions
- HPV 4 has ~100% efficacy against HPV16-related and HPV18-related vaginal and vulvar precancer lesions
- HPV4 has 99% efficacy against HPV6-related and HPV11-related genital warts in women
- HPV4 has 90% efficacy against HPV6-related and HPV11-related genital warts in men

Postmarketing surveillance in the United States, including data from the National Health and Nutrition Examination Surveys (NHANES), continues to show good efficacy for the HPV vaccines. Data comparing 2003 to 2006 with 2007 to 2010, the first 4 years of the HPV vaccination program in the United States, have shown the following[12]:

- Fifty-six percent reduction in prevalence of HPV types 6, 11, 16, and 18 in girls aged 14 to 19 years
- Thirty-six percent reduction in genital warts in US girls 15 to 19 years of age from 2006 to 2010

Surveillance across the globe in areas where 3-dose immunization rates in girls are 70% and higher shows even more promise:

- Seventy-five percent reduction in low-grade cervical abnormalities in Australian girls[13]
- Forty-five percent reduction in genital warts in girls aged 16 to 17 years in Demark[14]

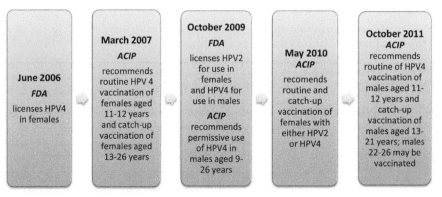

Fig. 1. HPV vaccination timeline. ACIP, Advisory Committee for Immunization Practices; FDA, US Food and Drug Administration.

Immunogenicity of Human Papillomavirus Vaccines

Immunogenicity studies for HPV4 have shown the following results[5]:

- Ninety-nine percent of girls had an antibody response to all 4 vaccine types 1 month after completing the 3-dose series
- Antibody response was higher in male patients and female patients aged 9 to 15 years compared with male patients and female patients aged 16 to 26 years
- At 36 months, seropositivity rates were 94%, 96%, 100%, and 76% to HPV6, HPV11, HPV16, and HPV18 respectively

Efficacy and Immunogenicity Data Summary

The HPV vaccine is efficacious against the included vaccine types. The best immune response with the HPV vaccine is seen in children aged 9 to 15 years, and excellent immunogenicity is seen for at least 10 years in girls and 5 years in boys after HPV vaccination.

ADOLESCENT VACCINATION RECOMMENDATIONS

The immunization guidelines are updated and revised continuously by the CDC, the ACIP, the Committee of Infectious Diseases of the American Academy of Pediatrics (AAP), and the American Academy of Family Physicians (AAFP).[15] **Table 3** summarizes the recommendations for the adolescent population.

The ACIP recommends administration of all age-appropriate vaccines during a single visit. HPV vaccination fits in well with other health recommendations for adolescents, which include anticipatory guidance about alcohol and smoking avoidance, as well as safer sex practices.

Table 4 shows the specifics of the HPV dosing and administration schedule.

Doses of HPV vaccine received at less than the recommended intervals should be readministered. If the HPV schedule is interrupted, the series does not need to be restarted. Whenever feasible, the same HPV vaccine should be used for the entire vaccination series. For best protection against HPV, adolescents should get all 3 doses of HPV vaccine before any sexual activity.

Indications and Contraindications for Human Papillomavirus Vaccination

Decisions on who should get the HPV vaccine are presented in **Table 5**.

Table 3
Recommended immunizations for adolescents

Vaccine	11–12 y	13–15 y	16–18 y
Tdap[a]	1 dose	Catch-up	Catch-up
Influenza	Annual vaccination		
HPV2, female patients only HPV 4, male and female patients	3-dose series	Catch-up	Catch-up
MCV4[b]	First dose	Catch-up	Booster dose

[a] Tdap: tetanus toxoid, reduced diphtheria toxoid, and acellular pertussis vaccine.
[b] MCV4: quadrivalent meningococcal conjugate vaccine.

Table 4
HPV vaccination schedule

	Recommended Vaccination Age (y)	Routine Vaccine Schedule	Catch-up Vaccine Schedule[a]
HPV 2	11–12	3-dose series at 0, 1–2[b], 6[c] mo	Administer at age 13–18 y if not previously vaccinated
HPV 4	11–12	3-dose series at 0, 1–2[b], 6[c] mo	Administer at age 13–18 y if not previously vaccinated

[a] Follow these routine dosing intervals for vaccine catch-up.
[b] Administer second dose 1 to 2 months after the first dose (minimum interval of 4 weeks.).
[c] Administer third dose 24 weeks after the first dose and 16 weeks after the second dose (minimum interval of 12 weeks between second and third doses).
Data from CDC. Advisory Committee on Immunization Practices recommended immunization schedules for persons aged 0 through 18 years – United States, 2014. MMWR Morb Mortal Wkly Rep 2014;63(5):108–9. Available at: http://www.cdc.gov/mmwr/preview/mmwrhtml/mm6305a6. htm. Accessed February 24, 2014.

Vaccine Coverage

Although most health insurance plans cover the HPV vaccine, it is best to check with individual carriers. The Vaccines for Children (VFC) program covers the cost of HPV vaccination for eligible uninsured and underinsured children younger than 19 years.[16]

Vaccine Costs

The cost for either vaccine ranges from $130 to $170 per dose, not including administration charges. The bill for the 3-dose series can exceed $500, making HPV one of the most expensive vaccines ever.[17]

Adolescent Vaccination Summary

HPV vaccination in a 3-dose series given over 3 months is recommended for routine use in all adolescents 11 to 12 years of age as part of comprehensive adolescent

Table 5
Deciding who should get the HPV vaccine

Who Should Get the Vaccine?	Who Should Wait?	Who Should Not Get the Vaccine?
Immunosuppressed teens[a] Teens with minor acute illnesses Lactating teens Teens with abnormal cervical cancer screenings[b] Teens with genital warts[c]	Pregnant teens[d] Teens with moderate or severe illnesses	Teens with life-threatening allergic reactions to any part of the vaccine or to a previous dose of vaccine[e]

[a] Immune response and vaccine efficacy may be less than those in immunocompetent adolescents.
[b] HPV vaccine is recommended to protect against HPV types not already contracted.
[c] HPV vaccine is recommended to protect against HPV types not already contracted.
[d] No safety concerns have been identified in the HPV pregnancy registry. Pregnancy testing before vaccination is not needed.
[e] HPV4 is produced in *Saccharomyces cerevisiae* (baker's yeast) and prefilled syringes of HPV2 have latex in the rubber stopper.
Data from CDC. Quadrivalent human papillomavirus vaccine, recommendations of the Advisory Committee on Immunizations Practices. MMWR Morb Mortal Wkly Rep 2007;56(RR02):1–24. Available at: http://www.cdc.gov/mmwr/preview/mmwrhtml/rr5602a1.htm. Accessed February 24, 2014.

health care. Most adolescents can receive the HPV vaccine, and the HPV vaccine is covered by most insurance carriers and the VFC program.

HUMAN PAPILLOMAVIRUS VACCINE SAFETY

From June 2006 to March 2013, ~57 million doses of HPV vaccine were distributed in the United States. With HPV4 comprising 99% of the doses distributed, analysis of vaccine safety is limited to HPV4. The CDC and FDA use several systems to monitor postlicensure vaccine safety, including[18]:

- Vaccine Adverse Event Reporting System (VAERS): a voluntary early warning system
- Vaccine Safety Datalink (VSD): collaborative effort with health care organizations to monitor adverse events

Overview of Vaccine Adverse Event Reporting System Findings

From June 2006 to March 2013, there were 21,194 adverse events received by VAERS, with reports declining significantly since peaking in 2008.[12]

- HPV4 adverse events are similar to those reported for other adolescent vaccines
- Nonserious or mild events represent 92.1% of the reports to VAERS
- Serious events (those resulting in hospitalization, prolongation of an existing hospitalization, permanent disability, life-threatening illness, or death) peaked in 2009 at 12.8% and have decreased steadily since
- No new or unusual patterns of adverse events suggest HPV vaccine safety concerns

Fig. 2 shows the proportion of serious and nonserious reports of adverse events after HPV vaccination reported to VAERS from June 2006 to March 2013. **Table 6** details the specific HPV-associated adverse events that have been reported to VAERS.

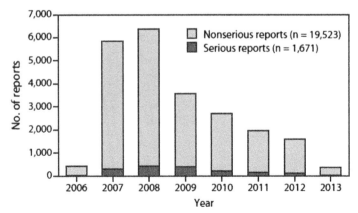

Fig. 2. The number of reports of serious and nonserious adverse events after administration of quadrivalent HPV (HPV4) vaccine in female patients, by year, in the United States from June 2006 to March 2013. Reporting peaked in 2008 and decreased each year thereafter; the proportion of reports to the VAERS that were classified as serious reports peaked in 2009 at 12.8% and decreased thereafter to 7.4% in 2013. (*From* CDC. Human papillomavirus vaccination coverage among adolescent girls, 2007-2012, and postlicensure vaccine safety monitoring, 2006-2013–United States. MMWR Morb Mortal Wkly Rep 2013;62(29):593.)

Table 6	
Adverse events associated with HPV vaccine in male and female patients as reported to VAERS	
Nonserious Adverse Events	**Serious Adverse Events**
Local adverse events	Headache
o Reactions at the injection site (97% mild to moderate)	Nausea
■ Pain (up to 9 in 10 patients)	Vomiting
■ Redness	Fatigue
■ Swelling	Dizziness
Systemic adverse events (most are mild to moderate)	Syncope
o Fever	Generalize weakness
■ Mild (37.8°C [100°F]) (1 in 10 patients)	
■ Moderate (38.9°C [102°F]) (1 in 65 patients)	
Other common side effects	
o Syncope	
o Headache	
o Dizziness	
o Nausea	
o Urticaria	
o Muscle or joint pain	

Data from FDA. Gardasil [package insert]. Available at: http://www.fda.gov/Biologics BloodVaccines/Vaccines/ApprovedProducts/ucm094042.htm. Accessed February 24, 2014.

Syncope

Adolescents may faint after medical procedures, including receiving shots. Syncope is described in 13% of VAERS reports pertaining to HPV4. This percentage is similar to reports of syncope for other adolescent vaccines. Of these reports, 15% resulted in a fall or injury. To prevent syncope-related injuries, providers are advised to take appropriate measures to prevent fainting and fainting-related injuries by following the ACIP recommendation to strongly consider observing patients for 15 minutes after vaccination.[19]

Other Postmarketing Surveillance

Continued safety surveillance has not shown an increase for any of the following conditions following HPV vaccination[20]:

- Guillain-Barré syndrome
- Stroke or venous thromboembolism
- Appendicitis
- Seizures
- Allergic reactions or anaphylaxis
- Ovarian failure

Deaths

Through 2013, there were 85 postvaccination deaths reported to VAERS, of which 43 were confirmed. There were no unusual patterns to the deaths suggesting that they were caused by the HPV vaccine.[20]

Safety Data Summary

Seven years of postlicensure safety monitoring in the United States provides continued evidence of the safety of HPV4. No new safety concerns have been identified in either male or female patients. Based on the available safety monitoring data, HPV vaccination continues to be recommended and its benefits continue to outweigh its risks.[21]

NATIONAL VACCINATION COVERAGE FOR ADOLESCENTS

Public education is an important first step after the introduction of a new vaccine. Providers also need time to accept new vaccines and to set up appropriate systems for their administration. Success of these steps is reflected in vaccination coverage rates. The CDC monitors vaccination coverage among adolescents aged 13 to 17 years with the National Immunization Survey–Teen (NIS-Teen.) **Fig. 3** represents 7 years of vaccine coverage in adolescents.[22]

Significant points from the NIS-Teen data are:

- From 2011 to 2012, vaccination coverage increased for Tdap, MCV4 (quadrivalent meningococcal conjugate vaccine), and HPV for male patients
- From 2011 to 2012, vaccination coverage for HPV for female patients decreased

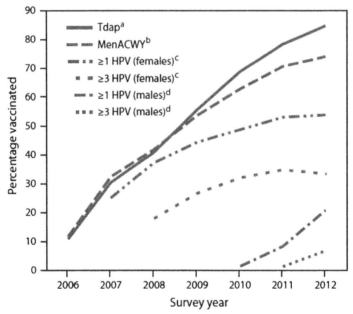

Fig. 3. Estimated vaccination coverage with selected vaccines and doses among adolescents aged 13 to 17 years, by survey year, from the National Immunization Survey–Teen, United States, 2006 to 2012. During 2007 to 2011, coverage for greater than or equal to 1 HPV vaccine dose among female patients lagged behind estimates for tetanus, diphtheria, acellular pertussis vaccine, and meningococcal conjugate vaccines, increasing on average 6.1 (95% confidence interval, 3.3–8.9) percentage points each year. However, in 2011 and 2012, HPV vaccination rates among female patients did not increase. [a] Greater than or equal to 1 dose of Tdap vaccine on or after age 10 years. [b] Greater than or equal to 1 dose MenACWY vaccine. [c] HPV vaccine, either bivalent or quadrivalent, among female patients. [d] HPV vaccine, either bivalent or quadrivalent, among male patients. ACIP recommends the quadrivalent vaccine for male patients. (*From* CDC. National and state vaccination coverage among adolescents aged 13-17 years–United States, 2012. MMWR Morb Mortal Wkly Rep 2012;62(34):687.)

- Coverage for greater than or equal to 1 HPV vaccine dose among female patients increased at a rate that lagged behind estimates for both Tdap and MCV4 vaccines
- First-year coverage for male patients was significantly lower than first-year coverage for female patients

Table 7 summarizes the NIS-Teen estimated vaccine coverage for all recommended vaccines in adolescents aged 13 to 17 years in 2011 to 2012.
Table 8 summarizes the NIS-Teen estimated HPV vaccine coverage among adolescent female patients aged 13 to 17 years, 2007 to 2012.

Key Points from the National Immunization Survey–Teen Data

- Coverage with Tdap and MCV4 vaccines has reached 85% and 74% respectively
- HPV vaccination for girls
  - Coverage with greater than or equal to 1 dose of any HPV vaccine increased from 25.1% in 2007 to 53.8% in 2012 but did not significantly increase from 2011 to 2012
  - Missed opportunity for HPV vaccination increased from 20.8% in 2008 to 84.0% in 2012
  - Completion of the 3-dose HPV vaccine series remained unchanged from 2011 to 2012
  - In girls between 13 and 17 years of age, ~50% have not started and ~33% have not completed the HPV vaccine series
- HPV vaccination for boys
  - Coverage increased significantly from 8.3% in 2011 to 20.8% in 2012; the first year after HPV vaccine was recommended for routine use in boys
  - Only 6.8% of boys aged 13 to 17 years have completed the HPV vaccine series

BARRIERS TO VACCINATION

Multiple strategies for increasing vaccination coverage in adolescents have been described in the literature, and achieving high vaccination rates is feasible. There

Table 7			
Vaccine coverage in adolescents, 2011 to 2012			
Vaccine	% in 2011 (n = 19,199)	% in 2012 (n = 23,564)	% Change
Tdap (≥1 dose)	78.2	84.6	+6.4
MCV4 (≥1 dose)	70.5	74.0	+3.5
HPV (1 dose)			
Female patients	53.0	53.8	+0.8
Male patients	8.3	20.8	+12.5
HPV (2 doses)			
Female patients	43.9	43.9	No change
Male patients	3.8	12.7	+8.9
HPV (3 doses)			
Female patients	34.8	33.4	−1.4
Male patients	1.3	6.8	+5.5

Data from CDC. National and state vaccination coverage among adolescents aged 13-17 years– United States, 2012. MMWR Morb Mortal Wkly Rep 2012;62(34):685–93. Available at: http:// www.cdc.gov/mmwr/preview/mmwrhtml/mm6234a1.htm. Accessed February 24, 2014.

Table 8
HPV vaccine coverage in female adolescents 2007 to 2012

	% in 2007	% in 2008	% in 2009	% in 2010	% in 2011	% in 2012
1 dose HPV	25.1	37.2	44.3	48.7	53.0	53.8
2 doses HPV	16.9	28.3	35.8	40.7	43.9	43.4
3 doses HPV	5.9	17.9	26.7	32.0	34.8	33.4
≥1 missed opportunity for HPV vaccine	20.8	30.8	52.5	67.9	77.7	84.0
Potential coverage with ≥1 HPV vaccine if no missed opportunity	40.6	56.5	73.5	83.5	89.5	92.6

Adapted from CDC. Human papillomavirus vaccination coverage among adolescent girls, 2007-2012, and postlicensure vaccine safety monitoring, 2006-2013–United States. MMWR Morb Mortal Wkly Rep 2013;62(29):591–5. Available at: http://cdc.gov/mmwr/preview/mmwrhtml/mm6229a4.htm. Accessed February 24, 2014.

are also additional barriers that require special attention with regard to HPV vaccination.[23]

NIS-Teen provides insight into some of the HPV vaccination barriers. The survey asks parents who did not intend to vaccinate their daughters in the next 12 months the primary reasons behind their decisions. In 2012, approximately one-quarter of surveyed parents did not intend to vaccination their daughters in the next 12 months. **Table 9** shows the top 5 parental responses for not vaccinating over the last 5 years.

Over the last 5 years, parental questions, concerns, and beliefs about HPV vaccination have continued to be significant barriers to increasing HPV vaccination rates for adolescents. The AAP Committee on Bioethics has provided several suggestions for approaching the management of parental hesitancy or refusal to vaccinate, focused on[24]:

- Establishing open and ongoing dialogue with families regarding their concerns
- Targeting education to address specific concerns raised using a variety of resources
- Maintaining the provider-patient relationship

Table 9
Top 5 reasons for not vaccinating adolescent daughters with HPV

Reason[a]	% in 2008	% in 2010	% in 2012	% Change Overall
Not needed or necessary	14.4	17.4	19.1	+4.7
Not recommended by provider	10.8	8.5	14.2	+3.4
Safety concerns/side effects	4.5	16.4	13.1	+8.6
Lack of knowledge about vaccine or disease	15.8	10.2	12.6	−3.2
Teen not sexually active	14.1	11.1	10.1	−4.0

[a] Response categories are not mutually exclusive.

Data from CDC. Human papillomavirus vaccination coverage among adolescent girls, 2007-2012, and postlicensure vaccine safety monitoring, 2006-2013–United States. MMWR Morb Mortal Wkly Rep 2013;62(29):591–5. Available at: http://cdc.gov/mmwr/preview/mmwrhtml/mm6229a4.htm. Accessed February 24, 2014; and Darden PM, Thompson DM, Roberts JR, et al. Reasons for not vaccinating adolescents: National Immunization Survey of Teens, 2008–2010. Pediatrics 2013;131(4):645–51.

Based on the NIS-Teen data, the following tips may also be useful in conversations with families and teens about HPV vaccination[25]:

- Frame HPV vaccines as vaccines that prevent cancers
- Provide factual information about HPV and HPV-associated health problems
- Address common myths, misconceptions, and misinformation about HPV vaccines
- Highlight the safety of HPV vaccines

Sex and the Human Papillomavirus Vaccine

A new study found no evidence that getting the HPV vaccine encourages young girls to engage in sexual activity or to start having sex at a younger age. Girls' beliefs about the HPV vaccine had no bearing on their decisions to become sexually active or to engage in risky sexual behaviors.[26]

The 1991 to 2011 Youth Behavioral Risk Surveys (YBRS) of 9th to 12th graders in the United States provides information to reinforce the importance of vaccination at the recommended ages of 11 to 12 years[27]:

- Half of all students report having ever been sexually active; including one-third of ninth graders
- Neither the percentage of all students who reported having ever been sexually active nor the percentage who reported having sex for the first time before the age of 13 years changed significantly after the introduction of the HPV vaccine

NOW IS THE TIME FOR ACTION: HUMAN PAPILLOMAVIRUS VACCINATION IN THE NATIONAL SPOTLIGHT

In 2012, only 33% of girls aged 13 to 17 years had received the recommended 3 doses of HPV vaccine. Current estimates are that 46,000 future cervical cancer cases over the lifetimes of girls younger than 12 years of age are being prevented by current levels of vaccination. For every year that coverage remains 30% rather than the target 80%, another 4400 girls will go on to develop cervical cancer.[6] The lack of progress with HPV vaccination among adolescents warrants action at a national level by health care providers, parents, public health agencies, and other immunization stakeholders.

Earlier this year, the 2012 to 2013 President's Cancer Panel report described HPV vaccination as "one of the most profound opportunities in cancer prevention today."[25] The panel, an advisory board of the National Cancer Institute (NCI), outlined 3 critical goals to accelerate HPV vaccine uptake in the United States.

- Reduce missed clinical opportunities to recommend and administer HPV vaccines
- Increase parents', caregivers', and adolescents' acceptance of HPV vaccines
- Maximize access to HPV vaccination services

On February 12, 2014, the leading medical and public health organizations, including the AAFP, the AAP, the American College of Physicians (ACP), and the American College of Obstetricians and Gynecologists (ACOG), along with the CDC and Immunization Action Coalition, released a Dear Colleague statement urging physicians in the United States to educate their patients about the HPV vaccine and to strongly encourage HPV vaccination. Their united message was: "What you say matters; how you say it matters even more."[28]

Areas to Be Addressed to Improve Human Papillomavirus Vaccination

1. Education of parents/guardians and adolescents
   - Three of the 5 reasons parents reported for not intending to vaccinate indicate gaps in understanding of both HPV disease and the HPV vaccine.
   - Updated educational materials for providers, parents and guardians, and adolescents are available from the CDC.[29]
2. Increase health care providers' consistency and strength of HPV vaccination recommendations
   - Individuals receiving a vaccine recommendation from a health care provider are significantly more likely to obtain an HPV vaccine than individuals who do not receive a recommendation.[28]
   - The CDC has developed a tips sheet to help providers respond to parents' questions and to communicate strong, clear HPV vaccination recommendations.[30]
3. Reduce missed opportunities to vaccinate
   - The CDC has comprehensive strategies to address a wide range of missed opportunities that providers may have in their own practices.[31]

SUMMARY

HPV vaccination is safe and effective against HPV-related diseases; it is cancer prevention. Despite this information, HPV vaccination rates are significantly less than those of other recommended adolescent vaccines. Providers who care for adolescents are urged to educate patients and adolescents about the HPV vaccine and to strongly recommend HPV vaccination as a 3-dose series for girls and boys 11 to 12 years of age as part of routine adolescent health care.

REFERENCES

1. CDC. Genital HPV infection fact sheet. Available at: http://www.cdc.gov/std/hpv/stdfact-hpv.htm. Accessed February 24, 2014.
2. CDC. CDC fact sheet: incidence, prevalence, and cost of sexually transmitted infections in the United States. 2013. Available at: http://www.cdc.gov/std/stats/STI-Estimates-Fact-Sheet-Feb-2013.pdf. Accessed February 24, 2014.
3. Dunne EF, Unger ER, Sternberg M, et al. Prevalence of HPV infection among females in the United States. JAMA 2007;297(8):876–8.
4. Centers for Disease Control and Prevention (CDC). Human papillomavirus-associated cancers–United States, 2004-2008. MMWR Morb Mortal Wkly Rep 2012;61(15):258–61. Available at: http://www.cdc.gov/mmwr/preview/mmwrhtml/mm6115a2.htm. Accessed February 24, 2014.
5. Centers for Disease Control and Prevention (CDC). Quadrivalent human papillomavirus vaccine, recommendations of the Advisory Committee on Immunizations Practices. MMWR Morb Mortal Wkly Rep 2007;56(RR02):1–24. Available at: http://www.cdc.gov/mmwr/preview/mmwrhtml/rr5602a1.htm. Accessed February 24, 2014.
6. AAP. HPV vaccine speaking points. 2013. Available at: http://www.aap.org/en-us/my-aap/advocacy/workingwiththemedia/speaking-tips/Pages/HPV-Vaccine.aspx. Accessed February 24, 2014.
7. CDC. Human papillomavirus (HPV). Making sense of your Pap & HPV test results. Available at: http://www.cdc.gov/sTd/hpv/pap/default.htm. Accessed February 24, 2014.

8. FDA. Gardasil. Available at: http://www.fda.gov/BiologicsBloodVaccines/Vaccines/ApprovedProducts/ucm094042.htm. Accessed February 24, 2014.

9. FDA. Cervarix. Available at: http://www.fda.gov/BiologicsBloodVaccines/Vaccines/ApprovedProducts/ucm186957.htm. Accessed February 24, 2014.

10. Centers for Disease Control and Prevention (CDC). FDA licensure of bivalent human papillomavirus vaccine for use in females and updated HPV vaccination recommendations from the Advisory Committee on Immunization Practices. MMWR Morb Mortal Wkly Rep 2010;59(20):626–9. Available at: http://www.cdc.goc/mmwr/preview/mmwrhtml/mm5920a4.htm. Accessed February 24, 2014.

11. Centers for Disease Control and Prevention (CDC). FDA licensure of quadrivalent human papillomavirus vaccine for use in males and guidance from the Advisory Committee on Immunization Practices. MMWR Morb Mortal Wkly Rep 2010;59(20):630–2. Available at: http://www.cdc.gov/mmwr/preview/mmwrhtml/mm5902a5.htm. Accessed February 24, 2014.

12. Centers for Disease Control and Prevention (CDC). Human papillomavirus vaccination coverage among adolescent girls, 2007-2012, and postlicensure vaccine safety monitoring, 2006-2013–United States. MMWR Morb Mortal Wkly Rep 2013;62(29):591–5. Available at: http://cdc.gov/mmwr/preview/mmwrhtml/mm6229a4.htm. Accessed February 24, 2014.

13. Ali H, Donovan B, Wand H, et al. Genital warts in young Australians five years into national human papillomavirus vaccination programme: national surveillance data. BMJ 2013;346:f2032.

14. Baandrup L, Blomberg M, Dehlendorff C, et al. Significant decrease in the incidence of genital warts in young Danish women after implementation of a national human papillomavirus vaccination program. Sex Transm Dis 2013;40:130–5.

15. Centers for Disease Control and Prevention (CDC). Advisory Committee on Immunization Practices recommended immunization schedules for persons aged 0 through 18 years – United States, 2014. MMWR Morb Mortal Wkly Rep 2014;63(5):108–9. Available at: http://www.cdc.gov/mmwr/preview/mmwrhtml/mm6305a6.htm. Accessed February 24, 2014.

16. CDC. HPV vaccine-questions & answers. Available at: http://www.cdc.gov/vaccines/vpd-vac/hpv/vac-faqs.htm. Accessed February 24, 2014.

17. American Cancer Society. Human papilloma virus (HPV), cancer, HPV testing, and HPV vaccines: frequently asked questions. Available at: http://www.cancer.org/cancer/cancercauses/othercarcinogens/infectiousagents/hpv/humanpapillomavirusandhpvvaccinesfaq/hpv-faq-vaccine-cost. Accessed February 24, 2014.

18. CDC. Vaccine safety human papillomavirus (HVP) vaccine. Available at: http://www.cdc.gov/vaccinesafety/Vaccines/HPV/Index.html. Accessed February 24, 2014.

19. Centers for Disease Control and Prevention (CDC). Syncope after vaccination — United States, January 2005–July 2007. MMWR Morb Mortal Wkly Rep 2008;57(17):457–60. Available at: http://www.cdc.gov/mmwr/preview/mmwrhtml/mm5717a2.htm. Accessed February 24, 2014.

20. Gee J, Naleway A, Shui I, et al. Monitoring the safety of quadrivalent human papillomatosis vaccine: findings from the vaccine safety datalink. Vaccine 2011;29(46):8279–84.

21. CDC. Frequently asked questions about HPV vaccine safety. Available at: http://www.cdc.gov/vaccinesafety/Vaccines/HPV/hpv_faqs.html. Accessed February 24, 2014.

22. Centers for Disease Control and Prevention (CDC). National and state vaccination coverage among adolescents aged 13-17 years–United States, 2012. MMWR

Morb Mortal Wkly Rep 2012;62(34):685–93. Available at: http://www.cdc.gov/mmwr/preview/mmwrhtml/mm6234a1.htm. Accessed February 24, 2014.

23. Darden PM, Thompson DM, Roberts JR, et al. Reasons for not vaccinating adolescents: National Immunization Survey of Teens, 2008-2010. Pediatrics 2013;131(4):645–51.

24. Diekema DS, American Academy of Pediatrics Committee on Bioethics. Responding to parental refusals of immunization of children. Pediatrics 2005; 115(5):1428–31.

25. National Cancer Institute. Accelerating HPV vaccine uptake: urgency for action to prevent cancer. A report to the President of the United States from the President's Cancer Panel. 2014. Available at: http://deainfo.nci.nih.gov/advisory/pcp/annualReports/HPV/index.htm. Accessed February 24, 2014.

26. Mayhew A, Kowalczyk M, Ding L, et al. Risk perceptions and subsequent sexual behaviors after HPV vaccination in adolescents. Pediatrics 2014;133(3):404–11.

27. Eaton DK, Kann L, Kinchen S, et al. Youth risk behavior surveillance–United States, 2011. MMWR Surveill Summ 2012;61(4):1–162.

28. AAP. Leading medical and public health organizations join efforts urging physicians to strongly recommend human papillomavirus (HPV) vaccination. 2014. Available at: http://www.aap.org/en-us/about-the-aap/aap-press-room/pages/Leading-Medical-and-Public-Health-Organizations-Join-Efforts-Urging-Physicians-to-Strongly-Recommend-Human-papillomavirus-.aspx. Accessed February 24, 2014.

29. CDC. Preteens and teens still need vaccines. Available at: http://www.cdc.gov/vaccines/who/teens/index.html. Accessed February 24, 2014.

30. CDC. Tips and time-savers for talking with parents about HPV vaccine. Available at: http://www.cdc.gov/vaccines/who/teens/for-hcp-tipsheet-hpv.html. Accessed February 24, 2014.

31. CDC. Assessment, feedback, initiatives, eXchange (AFIX) 2014 provider site visit questionnaire. 2014. Available at: www.cdc.gov/vaccines/programs/afix/site-visit-answers.pdf. Accessed February 24, 2014.

Evaluation and Management of Urinary Tract Infections in the School-Aged Child

G. Marcus Stephens, DO*, Scott Akers, DO, Hoa Nguyen, DO, Heidi Woxland, DO

KEYWORDS

- Pediatric urinary tract infection • Cystitis • Pyelonephritis • Vesicoureteral reflux

KEY POINTS

- Urinary tract infection (UTI) in the school-aged child is not uncommon.
- Unlike the younger child, who may present only with fever, the school-aged child usually has more typical symptoms of dysuria, frequency, or flank pain.
- *Escherichia coli* is still the most likely causative organism, and antibiotic therapy should empirically cover it until culture and sensitivity results are known.
- There is emerging antibiotic resistance by *E coli*, so local known sensitivity patterns may guide initial antibiotic choice. Third-generation and fourth-generation cephalosporins remain a good choice for most isolates.
- Voiding cystourethrography is no longer recommended after the first febrile UTI in the younger child.

INTRODUCTION AND OVERVIEW

The evaluation and management of urinary tract infection (UTI) in the school-aged child is an important part of primary care in the ambulatory setting. Acute UTIs are common in children. Guidelines regarding the diagnosis, treatment, and follow-up of UTIs in children continue to change. Although voiding cystourethrography (VCUG) is no longer recommended after the first febrile UTI in the younger child, it is important for primary care physicians to appropriately diagnose and treat UTIs in children. Renal scarring and renal disease, although rare, can lead to considerable morbidity later in life.

Disclosures: none.
Via Christi Family Medicine Residency, Department of Family Medicine, Kansas City University of Medicine and Biosciences, 707 North Emporia Street, Wichita, KS 67214, USA
* Corresponding author.
E-mail addresses: marc@stephens.net; marc.stephens@viachristi.org

Prim Care Clin Office Pract 42 (2015) 33–41
http://dx.doi.org/10.1016/j.pop.2014.09.007   **primarycare.theclinics.com**

EPIDEMIOLOGY

It is difficult to accurately obtain a reliable measure of the incidence of UTIs in children older than 2 years. Approximately 1% of boys and 3% to 5% of girls have at least 1 episode of UTI during childhood, and 30% to 50% of these children have at least 1 recurrence.[1]

When extending the age range and taking gender into account, European studies show that 10% of females and 3% of males have had a UTI before the age of 16 years.[2] Recurrence rates are as high as 30% to 50% in the United States and result in 1.5 million clinic visits annually.[1] Others estimate that these figures underrepresent numbers of UTIs, because most studies report only data that include a positive urine culture, rather than including those who have a high likelihood of UTI based on clinical suspicion and then are subsequently treated.[1] Furthermore, most studies fail to characterize UTIs as either complicated or uncomplicated, based on the presence of underlying anatomic or physiologic abnormalities within the urinary tract.[1] Uncomplicated cystitis is limited to the lower urinary tract segment and generally occurs in older children and adolescents, without any anatomic or physiologic abnormalities that predispose to a complicated UTI.

RISK FACTORS

Important risk factors must be considered. Sexual intercourse is one of the most important risk factors for development of infection in women.[3] Men have a lower incidence of UTI than women. Risk factors for men include uncircumcised penis and men who have sex with men or intercourse with an infected female.[4] Sexually active men are at increased risk but to a lesser extent than women. In the absence of these risk factors, a UTI in boys may be suggestive of anatomic or renal abnormalities and must be considered in the workup.

Aggressive therapy in the past was based on the idea of long-term sequelae after UTI, such as recurrent UTIs in association with vesicoureteral reflux (VUR), renal scarring, chronic kidney disease, and hypertension. Recent studies question the association of VUR and subsequent renal scarring, and an evidence-based approach to management needs to be addressed.[5] Renal scarring risk factors were evaluated, and the reported risk factors were age at diagnosis, sex, race/ethnicity, treatment delay, inflammatory indices, recurrent infections, and presence of VUR.[6]

CAUSE

Conditions favorable for UTI depend on the ability of the bacteria to adhere to the urinary tract and the host's ability to activate an immune response.[2] Uropathogenic bacteria originate from gut and perineal flora.[2] Bacteria often colonize the periurethral area and migrate into the bladder, sometimes via instrumentation such as a urinary catheter.[7] The most common bacterial cause of UTI is uropathogenic *Escherichia coli* (UPEC).[8,9] Other pathogens include *Klebsiella*, *Proteus mirabilis*, *Pseudomonas*, coagulase-negative *Staphylococcus*, and *Staphylococcus aureus*.[2] However, studies have shown that these less common pathogens do not have the virulence factors seen in UPEC. Their ability to cause UTIs depends on the host factors, such as immunocompromised status or abnormal anatomy, which leads to urinary stasis.[2] Most children with UTI do not have anatomic abnormalities.[2]

PATHOGENESIS

UPEC is the most common pathogen that causes UTI and asymptomatic bacteriuria in children.[8] The body keeps the urinary tract free of bacteria by flushing it with urinary flow and by response of the innate immune system.[2] Virulence factors of UPEC allow the pathogen to adhere and grow in the host. FimH is the most common gene in UPEC that helps with adhesion of the pathogen to the lining of urinary tract.[8] The PapEF gene helps with adherence of the bacteria to the epithelial lining via P fimbriae, which is the most essential step in the development of infection.[8] After adherence to the urinary tract, UPEC is able to release its toxins, the most common of which is α-hemolysin, which is an extracellular cytolytic protein found in 50% of UPECs.[8] The level of α-hemolysin in the blood correlates with the severity of infection.[8] UPEC also has multiple ways of acquiring iron from its host by way of the fyuA gene, which is a component of the iron-acquisition system.[8] With increased antibiotic use, there is also an increase in antibiotic resistance.[7] UPEC resistance to penicillin is well known, but resistance to trimethoprim/sulfamethoxazole (TMP/SMX) is also on the increase.[7] Also, the increase in methicillin-resistant *Staphylococcus aureus* and vancomycin-resistant enterococci bacteria has increased the severity of UTI.[7]

The severity of inflammatory response also depends not only on the release of toxin by the pathogen alone but also on the response of the host immune system. The host has an innate immune response by way of toll-like receptors, which activate the transcription factors, causing cytokine and interferon production.[2] The severity of damage is associated with the level of cytokine in the blood and urine.[2] The genetic difference in host immune systems could account for the clinical response to a urinary tract pathogen, as in development of UTI versus asymptomatic bacteriuria.[2] The severity of infection is increased in immunocompromised hosts, such as those with diabetes or human immunodeficiency virus or the very young, whose immune system has not fully developed, such as deficiency of IgA antibody.[7] Children who are toilet training are also at increased risk of UTI, because of change in habits of voiding and stooling, poor hygiene, and also the ability to hold urine.[7]

As mentioned earlier, most children with UTI do not have abnormal urinary tract anatomy. However, abnormalities in function or anatomy increase risk and severity of UTI. Patients with neuropathic bladder, in cases of spina bifida, myelomeningeocele, or other forms of spinal cord injury could cause inadequate bladder emptying, high-pressure storing, and voiding.[7] High-pressure storage could lead to secondary VUR and trabeculated bladder.[7] High-pressure voiding could cause bladder diverticulae.[7] Inadequate voiding leads to formation of bladder stones, which may become infected.[7] Poor drainage of urine is another host factor that could increase the risk of UTI, because flushing urine through the urinary tract is 1 way that the host could eliminate bacteria from the tract.[7] Obstruction of urine could happen anywhere along the ureter secondary to stones, strictures, ureteropelvic junction, or from a mass effect from a tumor.[2] Congenital causes of poor drainage could result from megaureter, ureterocele, or congenital aperistaltic ureter.[7]

CLINICAL PRESENTATION

In the preschool population, it is often difficult to diagnose a source of infection because of their decreased ability to communicate symptoms. Signs of an infection are nonspecific, and include fever, irritability, poor feeding, and listlessness. It is important to perform a thorough examination and workup to rule out other sources of infection, such as meningitis, upper respiratory infection, pneumonia, or gastroenteritis. However, the presence of another cause for fever does not rule out UTI, because these infections could occur concurrently.[10]

In the school-aged child, symptoms of UTI may be more apparent, and include dysuria, urinary urgency, urinary frequency, urinary incontinence, abdominal pain, suprapubic tenderness, and back or flank pain.[10] Acute cystitis usually presents with dysuria, urinary urgency, and frequency without significant fever, and there also be suprapubic tenderness. Pyelonephritis may present without any lower urinary tract symptoms, but with higher fever (>38.5°C) and with flank pain or tenderness. UTI is the most common cause of fever in healthy children presenting with a temperature greater than 40°C.[10]

Urethritis without cystitis may also present in the school-aged child, and non-infectious causes should be considered. This condition may present as dysuria without frequency or urgency. A thorough history and physical examination should elucidate most of these causes. Differential diagnoses include periurethral trauma, chemical or irritant vulvovaginitis, ulcerative diseases such as herpes, sexual abuse, or dermatitis.

CLINICAL EVALUATION

A thorough history and physical examination in children with suspected UTI are impor-tant in identifying risk for recurrence or increased severity of infection. Physical exam-ination should include vital signs, especially temperature and blood pressure. Children with increased blood pressure and history of recurrent UTI could likely already have renal scarring.[7] Growth parameters are also important and help to identify signs of failure to thrive in infants and younger children with chronic or recurrent infections.[10] Examine the back to look for signs of neurogenic bladder, such as spina bifida or myelomeningeocele.[10] Evaluate the genitalia to look for vulvovaginitis or any anatomic abnormalities, such as phimosis or labial adhesions.[10] Most of these conditions should have manifested well before the child reaches school age.

In the older child with recurrent UTI, some consideration should be given to the possibility of associated conditions like constipation or bladder dysfunction, which may prompt urologic consultation. Bladder dysfunction may include symptoms of urinary incontinence or voiding difficulties, usually after age 5 years, and after having obtained some level of urinary and bowel continence.

URINALYSIS

Obtaining a clean voided urine specimen in the school-aged child is usually less complicated than in the preschool child, who may not be toilet trained. Although urine culture is the gold standard, it usually requires at least 2 days for results, and therefore, initial clinical decisions can be based on the more rapid evaluation of the urine using a dipstick analysis and a microscopic examination. The urine should be examined and cultured as soon as possible, because a delay of even a few hours can obscure the results, producing both false-positive and false-negative results.

A dipstick analysis can detect the presence of leukocyte esterase and nitrites, which have good sensitivity and specificity, respectively. However, a negative dipstick does not rule out a UTI, so in a child with suspected UTI, urine culture is still necessary.

Microscopic urinalysis involves examining a centrifuged urine specimen under a microscope, looking for white blood cells (WBCs) and bacteria. A positive test for UTI is defined as 5 or more WBCs per high power field, or the presence of any bacteria. Again, because the sensitivity is not 100%, a urine culture is still warranted in the clinical setting of suspected UTI.

Urine culture and sensitivity remain the gold standard for diagnosing UTI. A single organism cultured from a clean-catch midstream urine specimen indicates a true UTI if more than 100,000 colony-forming units per mL grow out. Lesser amounts are required to diagnose UTI if the urine was obtained via suprapubic aspiration of the bladder, or via urinary catheterization, namely more than 1000 or 10,000 colonies per mL, respectively. Lower colony counts in symptomatic patients may be considered significant as well.

IMAGING

The purpose of imaging in the setting of a UTI is to identify children with an abnormal genitourinary tract, who require further management to prevent recurrent UTIs and renal scarring.[9,11] The 2007 National Institute for Health and Care Excellence (NICE) guidelines and 2011 American Academy of Pediatrics (AAP) guidelines no longer recommend a VCUG after the first febrile UTI. Instead, renal and bladder ultrasonography is the initial test of choice. The 2011 AAP guidelines recommend renal and bladder ultrasonography in any child 2 to 24 months old with a febrile UTI.[5,9] According to the NICE guidelines, the timing of ultrasonography depends on the age of the child and on the clinical situation, as outlined in **Table 1**.[5,12]

If any abnormalities are noted, such as hydronephrosis or renal scarring, or if there is suspicion for VUR or obstruction, a VCUG should be obtained. If ultrasonography is normal, no further imaging is needed at that time. If a child develops recurrent UTI, the AAP recommends obtaining a VCUG.[9] In the setting of recurrent UTI, NICE guidelines recommend VCUG in children younger than 6 months and a dimercaptosuccinic acid renal scan in children older than 6 months.[12]

TREATMENT

Management and choice of antimicrobial agent should take local resistance patterns into consideration and is ideally based on culture results and sensitivities. In addition, any underlying medical problems must be taken into account, such as being immunocompromised or any known anatomic abnormalities that may alter the treatment approach. Experts recommend treating with an antibiotic empirically for an uncomplicated UTI in children between 2 and 13 years of age, and for the drug to adequately cover *E coli*. A second-generation or third-generation cephalosporin can provide excellent coverage for most gram-negative pathogens in the urinary tract. When identified, it is important to note that gram-positive organisms such as *Enterococcus* and *Staphylococcus saprophyticus* are not covered by first-generation and second-generation cephalosporins. Amoxicillin or amoxicillin-clavulanate and even nitrofurantoin treat most community-acquired *Enterococcus*. TMP-SMX is recommended in isolates of *S saprophyticus*.[13]

E coli is increasingly becoming resistant to amoxicillin, amoxicillin-clavulanate, TMP-SMX, and first-generation cephalosporins.[14] As a class, fluoroquinolones are

Table 1			
Recommended imaging schedule			
Timing of Ultrasonography	**<6 mo Old**		**>6 mo Old**
During acute infection	Recurrent UTI Atypical UTI[a]		Atypical UTI[a]
Within 6 wk of infection	Respond well to treatment within 48 h		Recurrent UTI

[a] Atypical UTI is defined as those who are seriously ill or who have poor urine flow, abdominal or bladder mass, increased creatinine level, sepsis, failure to respond to appropriate antibiotics within 48 hours, infection with non-*E coli* organisms.

Adapted from Urinary tract infection in children: diagnosis, treatment, and long term management. NICE Clinical Guidelines, No. 54. National Institute for Health and Care Excellence; 2007.p. 18–19.

effective in the treatment of uncomplicated UTIs, particularly *S saprophyticus*, which is a common cause of UTI in sexually active women. However, safety has not been well studied with these medications in children, and fluoroquinolones are not recommended.[15]

DURATION OF THERAPY

For young children, adolescent males, and children with recurrent, febrile, or complicated UTI, treatment duration should be 7 to 14 days.[16] A meta-analysis review[13] evaluating treatment in children who are afebrile with a presumptive diagnosis of UTI concluded that children who were treated for 1 day or with a single dose of an antimicrobial had decreased cure rates when compared with children who were treated for 7 to 14 days. The cure rates for those treated for a duration of 2 to 4 days were similar to those treated for 7 to 14 days. For children with upper UTI/pyelonephritis who were 3 months or older, the recommended treatment is oral antibiotics for 7 to 10 days. If oral antibiotics cannot be used, treatment with an intravenous antibiotic, such as cefotaxime or ceftriaxone, for 2 to 4 days followed by oral antibiotics for a total duration of 10 days is recommended.[12]

A Cochrane analysis included 16 randomized controlled trials (RCTs), in which 1116 children were studied, and it was observed in 6 of these studies that a 10-day antibiotic treatment significantly increased the number of children free of persistent bacteriuria compared with single-dose therapy.[17,18]

Persistent bacteriuria at the end of treatment was reported in 24% of children receiving single-dose therapy compared with 10% of children who were randomized to 10-day therapy. However, there were no significant differences between these groups regarding persistent symptoms, recurrence after treatment or reinfection after treatment. To study the effect of antibiotics on renal parenchymal damage, compliance, development of resistant organisms, or adverse events, there were insufficient data to measure these parameters. Despite the inclusion of 16 RCTs, methodological weakness and small sample sizes made it difficult to conclude if any of the included antibiotics or regimens was superior to another.[17]

Table 2 shows the recommendations of the Clinical Practice Guidelines from the AAP regarding antimicrobial therapy.

VESICOURETERAL REFLUX AND PROPHYLAXIS

Medical treatment of VUR involves daily antibiotic administration. The thought behind this is straightforward, in that the resultant sterile urine that is refluxed does not cause an inflammatory response and therefore prevent renal scarring. The most commonly used agents are TMP-SMX or nitrofurantoin. Dosage recommendation is typically half to one-quarter of the usual therapeutic dose.[19] There are long-term consequences that must be considered when prolonged antibiotics are administered, such as bone marrow suppression, nausea and vomiting, abdominal discomfort, and antibiotic resistance.[19] A Cochrane analysis in 2011 evaluated the efficacy and harm of long-term antibiotic administration to prevent recurrent UTI in children. A total of 1557 children were selected, and comparison was made between placebo (no treatment) and antibiotic prophylaxis from 10 weeks to 12 months. The following is an excerpt from the conclusions of this Cochrane analysis:

> *Compared to placebo/no treatment, when all studies were included, antibiotics did not appear to reduce the risk of symptomatic UTI (RR 0.75, 95% CI 0.36 to 1.53) however when we evaluated the effects of antibiotics in studies with low*

Table 2	
Antimicrobial agents for treatment of UTIs	
Antimicrobial Agent	**Dosage**
Parenteral	
Ceftriaxone	75 mg/kg, every 24 h
Cefotaxime	150 mg/kg per day, divided every 6–8 h
Ceftazidime	100–150 mg/kg per day, divided every 8 h
Gentamicin	7.5 mg/kg per day, divided every 8 h
Tobramycin	5 mg/kg per day, divided every 8 h
Piperacillin	300 mg/kg per day, divided every 6–8 h
Oral	
Amoxicillin-clavulanate	20–40 mg/kg per day in 3 doses
TMP/SMX	6–12 mg/kg trimethoprim and 30–60 mg/kg sulfamethoxazole per day in 2 doses
Sulfisoxazole	120–150 mg/kg per day in 4 doses
Cefixime	8 mg/kg per day in 1 dose
Cefpodoxime	10 mg/kg per day in 2 doses
Cefprozil	30 mg/kg per day in 2 doses
Cefuroxime axetil	20–30 mg/kg per day in 2 doses
Cephalexin	50–100 mg/kg per day in 4 doses

Data from Subcommittee on Urinary Tract Infection, Steering Committee on Quality Improvement and Management, Roberts KB. Urinary tract infection: clinical practice guideline for the diagnosis and management of the initial UTI in febrile infants and children 2 to 24 months. Pediatrics 2011;128(3):602.

risk of bias, there was a statistically significant reduction (RR 0.68, 95% CI 0.48 to 0.95). The effect was similar in children with vesicoureteric reflux (VUR) (RR 0.65, 95% CI 0.39 to 1.07) compared to those without VUR (RR 0.56, 95% CI 0.15 to 2.12). There was no consistency in occurrence of adverse events. Three studies reported antibiotic resistance, showing a non-significant increased risk for resistance to the antibiotic in the active treatment groups (RR 2.4, 95% CI 0.62 to 9.26). Five studies (4 analysed, 367 children) compared one antibiotic with another but all compared different combinations or different outcomes and studies were not pooled. Two studies reported microbial resistance, nitrofurantoin having a significantly lower risk of resistance than cotrimoxazole (RR 0.54, 95% CI 0.31 to 0.92).[20]

The overall conclusion was that long-term use of antibiotics appeared to reduce the risk of repeat symptomatic UTI in children susceptible to UTI. However, the benefit is small, and the risk of microbial resistance must be considered.[20]

FOLLOW-UP AND PREVENTION

UTIs, particularly recurrent or those involving the upper tract, can cause renal scarring, with resultant hypertension, chronic kidney disease, proteinuria, or preeclampsia.[5] Those at greatest risk are patients who have recurrent UTIs, VUR, or abnormal anatomy.[5] Therefore, a first febrile UTI does not require follow-up or a test of cure. However, families should be advised to seek care with any febrile illness, urinary symptoms, nausea, vomiting, persistent irritability, or failure to thrive, because 8% to 30% of children experience reinfection.[2] These symptoms need to be evaluated for a UTI with urinalysis and urine culture and treated empirically until a negative urine culture results. In any child with a history of UTI, monitoring height, weight, and blood pressure is recommended.[2,21]

Patients with VUR are at higher risk of renal damage, and therefore, require further monitoring. If grade I to II VUR is identified, it is reasonable to offer surveillance, with counseling to seek immediate medical attention in any febrile illness or to treat with prophylactic antibiotics. In grade III to V VUR, antibiotic prophylaxis is recommended, with surgery if the patient fails this medical treatment. A yearly VCUG and renal ultrasonography should be obtained to monitor for renal scarring or spontaneous resolution of VUR. If further scarring is noted, treatment needs to be advanced to either antibiotic prophlyaxis or surgery if the patient is already on antibiotics.[22] If renal scarring is noted, blood pressure and proteinuria should be monitored yearly. Creatinine levels should be monitored yearly if bilateral renal scarring is present.[2]

Bowel and bladder voiding dysfunction, which includes incontinence, constipation, and ineffective emptying the bladder, is often associated with diagnosis of UTI in children. In all cases of UTI, with or without VUR, it is beneficial to evaluate for voiding dysfunction, because it is a risk for UTI and may secondarily cause VUR.[2,5] Bladder training, such as timed voiding or avoiding carbonated drinks and caffeine, can improve bladder function and may lead to resolution of UTI. Bowel voiding dysfunction, such as constipation, should be treated with laxatives. Treatment of voiding dysfunction may not only prevent recurrent UTIs but may also lead to resolution of VUR.[5]

Other preventive measures may have some benefit. Circumcision is associated with reducing the risk of UTI. The number needed to treat to prevent 1 UTI is 111 patients.[5] According to the AAP, the benefits outweigh the risks, and the AAP recommend encouraging circumcision but leaving the decision to the parents. The use of cranberry juice requires further investigation. In a small study, its use did not significantly decrease the risk of a UTI. Also, cranberry juice is associated with risk of diarrhea, dental caries, and obesity. Probiotics may be helpful to rid the gut of pathogenic flora, which may lead to fewer UTIs.[2]

SUMMARY

- The appropriate diagnosis and treatment of UTI in the school-aged child is important to avoid long-term renal sequelae.
- Older children and adolescents usually have symptoms of UTI that are more typical than infants and younger children, including dysuria, urgency, frequency in the case of acute cystitis, or fever and flank pain with pyelonephritis.
- Although dipstick and microscopic urinalysis can be supportive of the diagnosis of UTI, growth of a single type of bacteria on urine culture is the gold standard.
- E coli is the most frequent uropathogen, and is best treated with antibiotics that are known to cover it and account for local patterns of E coli bacterial resistance.
- VUR is still an important consideration, especially in recurrent UTI.
- The 2007 NICE guidelines and 2011 AAP guidelines no longer recommend a VCUG after the first febrile UTI. Instead, renal and bladder ultrasonography is the first test of choice.

REFERENCES

1. Copp HL, Shapiro DJ, Hersh AL. National ambulatory antibiotic prescribing patterns for pediatric urinary tract infection, 1998–2007. Pediatrics 2011;127: 1027–33.

2. Jadresic L. Urinary tract infections in children. Paediatr Child Health 2013:1–4. Available at: http://dx.doi.org/10.1016/j.paed.2013.11.002.
3. Hooton TM, Scholes D, Hughes JP, et al. A prospective study of risk factors for symptomatic urinary tract infection in young women. N Engl J Med 1996; 335(7):468–74.
4. Hooton TM, Stamm WE. Diagnosis and treatment of uncomplicated urinary tract infection. Infect Dis Clin North Am 1997;11(3):551–81.
5. Paintsil E. Update on recent guidelines for the management of urinary tract infections in children: the shifting paradigm. Curr Opin Pediatr 2013;25(1):88–94.
6. Cheng CH, Hang JF, Tsau YK, Lin TY. Nephromegaly is a significant risk factor for renal scarring in children with first febrile urinary tract infections. J Urol 2011;186: 2353–7.
7. Clark C, Kennedy A, Shortliffe L. Urinary tract infection in children: when to worry. Urol Clin North Am 2010;37(2):229–41.
8. Yun KW, Kim HY, Park HK, et al. Virulence factors of uropathogenic *Escherichia coli* of urinary tract infections and asymptomatic bacteriuria in children. J Microbiol Immunol Infect 2013. http://dx.doi.org/10.1016/j.jmii.2013.07.010.
9. Roberts K. Revised AAP guideline on UTI in febrile infants and young children. Am Fam Physician 2012;86(10):940–6.
10. Hoberman A, Shaikh N. Urinary tract infections in infants and children older than one month: clinical features and diagnosis. UpToDate 2014.
11. Shaikh N, Hoberman A. Urinary tract infections in children: acute management, imaging, and prognosis. UpToDate 2014.
12. Urinary tract infection in children: diagnosis, treatment, and long term management. NICE Clinical Guidelines, No. 54. National Institute for Health and Clinical Excellence; 2007.
13. Tran D, Muchant DG, Aronoff SC. Short-course versus conventional length antimicrobial therapy for uncomplicated lower urinary tract infections in children: a meta-analysis of 1279 patients. J Pediatr 2001;139(1):93.
14. Prais D, Straussberg R, Avitzur Y, et al. Bacterial susceptibility to oral antibiotics in community acquired urinary tract infection. Arch Dis Child 2003;88(3):215–8.
15. Bradley J, Jackson M. The use of systemic and topical fluoroquinolones. Pediatrics 2011;128(4):e1034–45.
16. Subcommittee on Urinary Tract Infection, Steering Committee on Quality Improvement and Management, Roberts KB. Urinary tract infection: clinical practice guideline for the diagnosis and management of the initial UTI in febrile infants and children 2 to 24 months. Pediatrics 2011;128(3):595–610.
17. Fitzgerald A, Mori R, Lakhanpaul M, et al. Antibiotics for treating lower urinary tract infection in children. Cochrane Database Syst Rev 2012;(8):CD006857.
18. Practice parameter: the diagnosis, treatment, and evaluation of the initial urinary tract infection in febrile infants and young children. American Academy of Pediatrics. Committee on Quality Improvement: Subcommittee on Urinary Tract Infection. Pediatrics 1999;103(4 Pt 1):843–52.
19. Uhari M, Nuutinen M, Turtinen J. Adverse reactions in children during long-term antimicrobial therapy. Pediatr Infect Dis J 1996;15(5):404–8.
20. Williams G, Craig JC. Long-term antibiotics for preventing recurrent urinary tract infection in children. Cochrane Database Syst Rev 2011;(3):CD001534.
21. Shaikh N, Hoberman A. Urinary tract infections in children: long-term management and prevention. UpToDate 2014.
22. McLorie G, Herrin J. Management of vesicoureteral reflux. UpToDate 2014.

Childhood Cancer for the Primary Care Physician

Mohamed Radhi, MD[a],*, Joy M. Fulbright, MD[b], Kevin F. Ginn, MD[c],
Erin M. Guest, MD[a]

KEYWORDS

- Childhood cancer • Acute leukemia • Lymphoma • CNS tumors • Bone tumors
- Sarcoma • Wilms tumors • Risk factors

KEY POINTS

- Childhood cancer is rare among childhood diseases; however, it is a leading cause of death in children.
- Childhood cancer is a challenging disease entity because of its rarity, and it often presents with symptoms that overlap with more common, benign diseases.
- Childhood cancer can present at any age or in any organ.
- Although childhood cancer is usually a random event, it can be predisposed by certain genetic, familial, or immunologic disorders. Physicians need to have a general knowledge about these disorders so that they have an increased level of suspicion for cancer in these patients.
- Childhood cancer can be a life-threatening medical emergency that requires immediate and swift action to prevent loss of life.

INTRODUCTION

Childhood cancer is rare among childhood diseases. Despite being a rare disease entity in children, approximately 10,000 to 15,000 new cases per year of cancer occur in the first 2 decades of life in the United States.[1] Before they reach adulthood, 1 child in every 600 develops some type of childhood cancer, which is a principal cause of death in children.[1–4] Despite being a leading cause of death, survival of childhood cancer is much higher than that of adult cancer and is improving over time.[5] Making

Disclosures: None.
Conflict of interest: None.
[a] Division of Pediatric Hematology/Oncology/Bone Marrow Transplant, Children's Mercy Hospital, 2401 Gillham Road, Kansas City, MO 64108, USA; [b] Survive & Thrive Program, Division of Pediatric Hematology/Oncology/Bone Marrow Transplant, Children's Mercy Hospital, 2401 Gillham Road, Kansas City, MO 64108, USA; [c] Neuro-Oncology Program, Division of Pediatric Hematology/Oncology/Bone Marrow Transplant, Children's Mercy Hospital, 2401 Gillham Road, Kansas City, MO 64108, USA
* Corresponding author.
E-mail address: maradhi@cmh.edu

Prim Care Clin Office Pract 42 (2015) 43–55
http://dx.doi.org/10.1016/j.pop.2014.09.006 **primarycare.theclinics.com**

the diagnosis of childhood cancer can be challenging in the primary care setting. This difficulty may be caused by the vagueness of the presenting signs and symptoms of childhood cancer, the rarity of the cancer in childhood compared with adulthood, and the low index of suspicion that primary care providers have when dealing with such nonspecific symptoms.[3,4,6] The mean time of delay in diagnosis was found in one large review of 23 studies of childhood cancer to range from as short as 2.5 weeks for neuroblastoma to almost 30 weeks for brain tumors. This article about common childhood cancers discusses the cancers commonly encountered by general practitioners, focusing on key points that can help physicians recognize cancer early in the diagnostic process.

ACUTE LEUKEMIA
Epidemiology

Acute leukemia in children is categorized into 2 major disease types: acute lymphoblastic leukemia (ALL) and acute myeloid leukemia (AML), based on the phenotype of the leukemia blast cells. ALL is the most common cancer in children in the United States, accounting for 26% of new cancer diagnoses in the birth to 14-year age group and 2670 new cases per year.[7] ALL is more common in boys than in girls and in Hispanic and white children than in African American children. The peak incidence of ALL is among children aged 2 to 4 years. AML occurs in approximately 500 children in the United States per year, with the peak incidence in children less than 2 years old.[7] In the United States, survival rates of pediatric leukemia have improved over the past few decades, and now most children treated for leukemia survive without disease recurrence.

Clinical Presentation

Signs and symptoms of acute leukemia in children include fever (61% of cases), bone pain, lymphadenopathy, hepatomegaly, splenomegaly, pallor, bruising, and petechiae.[1] Bone pain may manifest in a young child as a limp or refusal to walk.[8] Constitutional symptoms, such as anorexia, weight loss, and fatigue, are also common. Complete blood count (CBC) findings may include leukocytosis or leukopenia (commonly neutropenia), anemia, and/or thrombocytopenia. Leukemia blast cells may be seen on the peripheral blood smear, but the absence of circulating blasts does not rule out acute leukemia. Other possible manifestations of acute leukemia include respiratory compromise secondary to a mediastinal mass; tumor lysis syndrome resulting in hyperuricemia, hyperkalemia, hyperphosphatemia, and acute kidney injury; opportunistic infections; disseminated intravascular coagulation (DIC); extramedullary infiltration of leukemia blasts into the skin or other soft tissues; and central nervous system (CNS) symptoms such as cranial nerve palsies and headaches.[9]

Differential Diagnosis

In the absence of blasts on the peripheral blood smear, the differential diagnosis should include infectious causes, autoimmune disease, and other malignancies. Lymphoma may present with features similar to acute leukemia. Neuroblastoma may also manifest with symptoms suggestive of leukemia, secondary to metastatic infiltration of the malignant cells into the bone marrow, liver, and bones.

Initial Diagnostic Work-up

Complete physical examination, with attention to vital sign stability, lymph nodes, liver and spleen size, skin, testes, and neurologic signs, is important at baseline. Initial laboratory testing should include a CBC with differential, pathology review of the peripheral blood smear, comprehensive metabolic panel, uric acid, serum phosphorus, lactate dehydrogenase (LDH), prothrombin time, partial thromboplastin time, and fibrinogen level. A chest radiograph should be performed to assess for a mediastinal mass. The patient should be referred to a pediatric oncologist for further work-up or, if unstable, the patient should be evaluated in an acute care facility. **Table 1** lists red flags, or signs and symptoms that warrant referral to a pediatric oncologist for suspected malignancy.

LYMPHOMA
Epidemiology

Lymphomas are classified broadly as either non-Hodgkin lymphoma (NHL) or Hodgkin lymphoma (HL). In children, the incidence of NHL is 620 cases per year in the United States and the most common subtypes are Burkitt lymphoma, diffuse large B-cell lymphoma, lymphoblastic lymphoma, and anaplastic large cell lymphoma.[7] Although HL occurs most commonly in adolescents, it is diagnosed in 380 children per year in the United States.[7]

Clinical Presentation

Lymph nodes in the cervical and axillary regions greater than 1.0 cm, inguinal region greater than 1.5 cm, or epitrochlear region greater than 0.5 cm are abnormal, but most often benign. Enlarged nodes that are firm, fixed to underlying tissue, and not associated with a known infection should prompt evaluation for lymphoma.[10] The challenge in children is that lymphadenopathy is a common examination finding, whereas malignant lymphoma is rare.[11] Therefore, consideration should be given to the size of the abnormal node, duration of the adenopathy, response to antibiotic treatment, and associated constitutional symptoms, such as the B symptoms of weight loss, fever, and night sweats. Children with mediastinal lymph node masses may present with dyspnea, cough, or orthopnea secondary to airway compression and require emergent evaluation.

Differential Diagnosis

Lymphadenopathy in a school-aged child is most commonly secondary to viral (eg, Epstein-Barr virus [EBV]) or bacterial infection. The differential is large and includes fungal, mycobacterial, and other more rare infectious causes, leukemia, solid tumors with metastases, immunologic diseases, and vasculitis.[10]

Initial Diagnostic Work-up

Complete physical examination, with documentation of all enlarged or otherwise abnormal nodes, testicular examination, liver and spleen size, and respiratory status should be performed. Initial laboratory testing is the same as in leukemia, assessing for bone marrow involvement with a CBC with differential and for tumor lysis syndrome with the comprehensive metabolic panel, uric acid, serum phosphorus, and LDH. EBV antibody titers and evaluation for other infectious causes should be considered. A chest radiograph is critical to evaluate for a mediastinal mass in patients with cervical, supraclavicular, or suprasternal adenopathy, even in the absence of respiratory symptoms. Fine-needle aspiration (FNA) may detect lymphoma, but excisional biopsy should be pursued if FNA is nondiagnostic and malignancy is strongly suspected.[12]

Table 1
Common childhood malignancies and associated clinical red flags that should prompt work-up by a pediatric oncologist

Malignancy	History/Symptom	Sign
Acute leukemia (ALL, AML)	Fever Pallor Bone pain or limp Infection (particularly of an unusual location, severity, or organism) Anorexia, weight loss Fatigue Bruising Petechiae Mucosal bleeding Dyspnea Orthopnea Headache Double vision	Fever Anemia WBC abnormalities (eg, leukocytosis, peripheral blasts, leukopenia, neutropenia) Lymphadenopathy, generalized Hepatosplenomegaly Thrombocytopenia DIC Gingival hypertrophy Mediastinal mass Pleural effusion Cranial nerve palsy
Lymphoma (NHL, HL)	Lymph node swelling Fever Weight loss Night sweats Pruritus Bruising Petechiae Cough Dyspnea Orthopnea Pain	Lymphadenopathy (nodes enlarged, firm, fixed, nontender) Fever Cytopenias (if bone marrow involvement) Hepatosplenomegaly Mediastinal mass Abdominal mass Intussusception
CNS tumors	Headache Vomiting Vision changes Irritability Weakness Loss of coordination Loss of developmental milestones Declining school performance	Cranial nerve palsy Neurologic deficits (ie, weakness, sensory loss) Ataxia Papilledema Parinaud (ie, paralysis of upward gaze) Full anterior fontanelle Abnormally increasing head circumference Seizures
Neuroblastoma	Enlarging abdomen Anorexia Weight loss Pallor Bruising Petechiae Bone pain Fever Irritability Diarrhea or constipation Back pain	Abdominal mass Posterior chest mass Cytopenias Periorbital bruising (raccoon eyes) Proptosis Opsoclonus myoclonus ataxia syndrome Horner syndrome Bony masses Hypertension Weakness or paralysis

(continued on next page)

Table 1		
(continued)		
Malignancy	**History/Symptom**	**Sign**
Wilms tumor	Enlarging abdomen	Abdominal mass
	Hematuria	Hematuria, gross or microscopic
	Constipation	Hypertension
	Abdominal pain	
Bone sarcoma	Bone pain	Palpable mass
(osteosarcoma,	Deformity	Deformity
Ewing sarcoma)	Swelling	Swelling
	Anorexia, weight loss	Pathologic fracture
	Symptoms caused by mass	Pulmonary nodules
	effect (eg, constipation from	
	pelvic tumor)	
Soft tissue sarcoma	Palpable mass	Palpable mass
(rhabdomyosarcoma	Deformity	Deformity
and other rare	Swelling	Various, depending on location
sarcomas)	Pain	of tumor
	Symptoms caused by mass	
	effect	

Abbreviations: HL, Hodgkin lymphoma; NHL, non-Hodgkin lymphoma; WBC, white blood cell.
  Data from Bernbeck B, Wuller D, Janssen G, et al. Symptoms of childhood acute lymphoblastic leukemia: red flags to recognize leukemia in daily practice. Klin Padiatr 2009;221(6):369–73; and Fragkandrea I, Nixon JA, Panagopoulou P. Signs and symptoms of childhood cancer: a guide for early recognition. Am Fam Physician 2013;88(3):185–92.

CENTRAL NERVOUS SYSTEM TUMORS
Epidemiology

Pediatric CNS tumors represent the second most common oncology diagnosis, the most common solid tumor, and a leading cause of cancer-related death.[13] Data from the Central Brain Tumor Registry of the United States (CBTRUS) from 2005 to 2009 showed an incidence of malignant CNS tumors of 3.3 per 100,000 for children 0 to 19 years of age and a nonmalignant CNS tumor incidence of 1.9 per 100,000.[14] Concerns continue regarding the possibility that the incidence of CNS tumors is increasing in the United States, with a recent review of SEER (Surveillance, Epidemiology, and End Results) data showing average annual increase of 1.37%.[15]

Clinical Presentation

Diagnostic delay has been reported to be associated with disseminated disease and decreased survival in some patients,[16,17] highlighting the importance of prompt diagnosis. Pediatric CNS tumors most commonly arise in the posterior fossa,[14] can appear throughout the CNS, and their symptoms correlate with location. Headache, nausea/vomiting, symptoms of hydrocephalus, and gait disturbances are the most common presentation in the emergency department.[18] Papilledema and seizures are also common at presentation.[19] Symptoms may initially be misdiagnosed as viral gastroenteritis, otitis media, sinus infection, migraine, or developmental/behavioral problems and follow-up of persistent symptoms is important. Patients may not present with classic early morning headache, but this should always raise suspicion.

Patients can deteriorate rapidly with obstructive hydrocephalus, leading to death[20–22] or permanent disability with spinal cord compression. Infants may have minimal symptoms, irritability, or increased head circumference as a primary presentation.

Spinal cord tumors are much less common and initial symptoms may include chronic back pain, neuropathic pain, difficulty walking, sensory changes, and eventually sphincter dysfunction and paralysis. One-third of patients with spinal cord tumors may have scoliosis.[23]

Differential Diagnosis

The symptoms associated with brain tumors may be dramatic, as is often the case with obstructive hydrocephalus, or subtle, such as abnormally increased head circumference in an infant. When obvious neurologic findings are not present, the differential diagnosis may be broad and may initially suggest a non-CNS cause. Once a tumor is identified on brain imaging, the differential becomes more focused. A brain neoplasm may be malignant or nonmalignant, although even a benign tumor can have serious consequences for the patient. Metastatic tumors from an extracranial cancer must be considered, although this is more common in adults. Infectious causes such as abscesses or fungal lesions of the brain are possible in children. Cavernous malformations,[24] arteriovenous malformations,[25] and congenital malformations[26] may lead to seizure and/or neurologic changes and mimic tumor on imaging. Rare causes like Rosai-Dorfman[27] or Langerhans cell histiocytosis (LCH)[28] should be considered, especially with diabetes insipidus and pituitary stalk changes, which are often seen with LCH.

Spinal cord tumors may occur in the extradural or intradural space. An extradural spinal cord tumor may represent leukemia or lymphoma, a bony vertebral tumor, or neuroblastoma.[29] Intradural extramedullary tumors include meningioma, myxopapillary ependymoma, peripheral nerve sheath tumors, and dermoid/epidermoid tumors.[23] Metastatic disease and infection must also be considered.

Initial Diagnostic Work-up

A detailed history and neurologic examination may localize the tumor before imaging. MRI is the modality of choice and baseline brain and spine imaging should be obtained in all new patients. Computed tomography (CT) scan may be obtained for rapid evaluation of hydrocephalus or hemorrhage.

History of urine output and baseline electrolytes should be considered because of the high risk of diabetes insipidus.[30]

Extracranial metastasis is rare. Bone, bone marrow, lymph nodes, lung, and liver are the most common sites. Bone pain or abnormal CBC should prompt investigation.[31]

Germ cell tumors are common in the suprasellar and pineal region. Serum alpha-fetoprotein and beta human chorionic gonadotropin should be obtained for tumors in these regions.[32]

NEUROBLASTOMA
Epidemiology

Neuroblastoma is the most common extracranial solid tumor of childhood. It accounts for about 10% for all childhood tumors with about 600 to 800 new cases per year, giving it a prevalence of 1 in 7000 live births.[1,33,34] Incidence peaks in the first 5 years of life with a median age of 22 months, and 95% of cases are diagnosed by 10 years of age.[33,35] Some cases of neuroblastoma regress spontaneously or they can even mature and become the more benign counterpart, ganglioneuroma. Most patients with stage 1 tumors require surgery only for cure.

Clinical Presentation

Most neuroblastomas arise in the abdominal cavity. However, thoracic tumors are more common in infants. About 1% of all neuroblastoma do not have an identifiable site of origin.[1] The signs and symptoms of neuroblastoma are mainly caused by the location and the extent of the primary disease and metastases. Low-stage localized disease is usually asymptomatic and disease is usually discovered with testing for unrelated medical conditions.[33,34] High cervical thoracic tumors usually present with Horner syndrome (unilateral ptosis, miosis, and anhidrosis), whereas large thoracic tumors can be associated with mechanical venous obstruction and a true superior vena cava syndrome (cough, dyspnea, facial edema/discoloration, and dysphagia). Orbital metastatic disease can present with periorbital bruising, commonly referred to as raccoon eyes, which can initially raise suspicion for child abuse.[34] Some of the other well-known clinical syndromes with which neuroblastoma can present include Pepper syndrome (massive involvement of the liver), Hutchinson syndrome (limping and irritability caused by bone and bone marrow metastasis), opsoclonus-myoclonus ataxia syndrome (paraneoplastic movement disorder), and Kerner-Morrison syndrome (intractable secretary diarrhea caused by vasoactive intestinal peptide secretion).[1]

Differential Diagnosis

Because of the many clinical syndromes, multiorgan involvement, and the variety of metastatic sites that can be involved with neuroblastoma, the differential diagnosis should include other neoplastic, in addition to nonneoplastic, conditions. Some of the nonmalignant conditions that can mimic neuroblastoma include inflammatory diseases such as osteomyelitis, inflammatory bowel disease, and rheumatoid arthritis. Multicystic or storage disorders should also be considered in patients with hepatomegaly.[1]

Initial Diagnostic Work-up

Population-based screening for increased catecholamine metabolite levels in children up to 1 year of age has considered and trialed, with the goal to detect the presence of neuroblastoma at an earlier stage. However, 2 large screening studies failed to show the effectiveness of such improvement in survival, despite increasing the incidence of neuroblastoma diagnosis, because a large proportion of these tumors can show maturation and never progress to malignancy.[1,36,37] Although most neuroblastoma cases are sporadic, recent data show that there is a small subgroup of familial cases with somatic mutation in the *ALK* or *PHOX2B* oncogenes. These patients may have a family history of neuroblastoma, Hirschsprung disease, or congenital central hypoventilation syndrome.[38]

In any child suspected of having neuroblastoma, a detailed examination including abdominal and lymph node assessment should be done. The head-and-neck evaluation should include assessment for proptosis and Horner syndrome. A full neurologic examination should also be documented. If a patient has a paraspinal mass, it is important to ensure that evolving paralysis is not missed. Definitive neuroblastoma diagnosis is confirmed by either unequivocal pathologic confirmation from evaluation of tumor tissue or by confirmation of neuroblastoma tumor cells in a bone marrow sample in the setting of increased urine or serum catecholamine levels.[1,33,34]

WILMS TUMOR
Epidemiology

Wilms tumor is the most common cause of malignant renal tumors of childhood. It is responsible for most (500 cases per year) renal tumors diagnosed in the United States. Only in patients aged 15 to 19 years is its incidence surpassed by clear cell carcinoma of the kidney.[1] The median age of presentation is about 3 years for boys and 4 years for girls, with higher incidence in African American children than in white children.[39]

Clinical Presentation

Most patients present with an abdominal mass that is typically asymptomatic and incidentally found while a caregiver is bathing the child. Abdominal examination should include careful evaluation for signs of venous obstruction like leg swelling, varicocele, or a distended abdominal wall.[39] Pain is the second most common symptom, followed by hematuria that is usually microscopic. However, macroscopic hematuria can occur and may indicate a large tumor.[1,40] One of the unique aspects of Wilms tumor is its association with a variety of familial syndromes and conditions. These associations have now been reported for almost 50 years.[41,42] Scott and colleagues[43] reported on 50 different syndromes and constitutional abnormalities that could be associated with Wilms tumor, and these were classified into high-risk, intermediate-risk, and low-risk conditions based on the incidence of Wilms tumor in each group. However, conclusive evidence to support mass screening of patients with these syndromes could not be made.

Differential Diagnosis

Wilms tumor must be differentiated from other primary malignancies of the kidney and from metastatic malignant tumors that involve the kidney, such as leukemia, Burkitt lymphoma, and sarcomas. Wilms tumor should also be differentiated from benign renal tumors, such as cystic disease of the kidney, hydronephrosis, or even a cold renal abscess. Collaborative international trials have shown that up to 10% of patients with preoperative diagnosis of Wilms had a different diagnosis.[44,45]

Initial Diagnostic Work-up

Initial laboratory work-up for kidney tumors should include a CBC, liver and renal function tests, urinalysis, and basic chemistries. To reduce the risk of preoperative tumor rupture, care should be taken not to aggressively examine the patient's abdomen, or to allow multiple examiners to palpate the tumor beyond what is medically necessary. Preoperative CT scan is the most accurate imaging technique for evaluation and is the best modality to detect lung metastasis.[1,39] Imaging should include assessment of the opposite kidney to determine whether bilateral Wilms tumors are present before surgical planning.

BONE AND SOFT TISSUE SARCOMA
Epidemiology

Osteosarcoma, with an incidence of 5 per million in persons aged 0 to 19 years, has a bimodal peak in adolescents and older adults.[1] It has a higher incidence in male patients and in African American and Hispanic populations. Osteosarcoma is associated with an *RB1* gene mutation, so patients with history of retinoblastoma (especially those diagnosed before 1 year of age) are at increased risk of developing osteosarcoma. Previous radiation therapy also increases the risk for developing osteosarcoma.[46] Ewing sarcoma has a higher incidence in white people than in other races, and an incidence of 2.9 cases per million.[1] Soft tissue sarcomas are classified as rhabdomyosarcoma and nonrhabdomyosarcoma and account for about 7% of childhood cancers in children and adolescents.[1]

Clinical Presentation

Bone pain that is not mechanical in nature is concerning in a child and could indicate infection or malignancy. When pain is the main presenting symptom (compared with more rare symptoms) there is often a longer delay until the diagnosis of cancer is made.[47] Suspicion should be raised if pain lasts longer than 3 weeks, is getting worse, or wakes a child up at night. Pathologic bone fracture may be the first presenting sign in a mass that was previously painless. A mass that is larger than 5 cm (golf ball size; ie, 42.58 mm in diameter), deep to fascia, increasing in size, and/or painful should be considered malignant until proved otherwise.[48] Other symptoms may also occur if the tumor is causing mass effect, such as superior vena cava syndrome, spinal cord compression, or proptosis.

Differential Diagnosis

Bone pain can be caused by a variety of mechanisms. Pain caused by trauma, mechanical overuse, osteochondrosis, and toxic synovitis are more common diagnoses than cancer in pediatrics. A soft tissue mass that fluctuates in size is often a fluid-filled bursa or ganglia.

Initial Diagnostic Work-up

Full physical examination and clinical history are essential to establish the differential diagnosis. A specific focus on lymph nodes, perfusion, neurologic status, and palpation of masses should be part of the physical examination. Length of symptoms, how they have progressed over time, and family/personal history of cancer are important historical points. A CBC with differential should be performed to evaluate for leukemia or bone marrow infiltration by other tumors. LDH and alkaline phosphatase are nonspecific markers of bone and soft tissue cell turnover and may suggest malignancy if their levels are significantly increased.

If the presenting symptom is bone pain without a palpable mass, then plain films, with at least 2 views in perpendicular, should be obtained of the site. Plain films can help guide the rest of the work-up and evaluate for fractures. Ultrasonography may differentiate between a fluid-filled versus a solid mass and should be used to evaluate suspicious scrotal masses. If initial testing is negative, but symptoms continue, then the patient should undergo MRI or CT scan of the site. MRI is preferred because it provides more soft tissue detail than CT.

A pediatric patient with a suspicious soft tissue mass or bone tumor should be referred to an orthopedic sarcoma surgeon or pediatric hematologist/oncologist before obtaining a biopsy. It is essential that the approach to biopsy is carefully considered because all of the tissues contaminated by the biopsy and its tract must later be removed during definitive therapy.[49]

RISK FACTORS FOR CANCER IN CHILDREN

Although most children who develop cancer have no known risk factors for malignant disease, certain children are at increased risk. Conditions that may predispose children to cancer include certain viral infections, immunodeficiency, genetic syndromes, prematurity and low birth weight (associated with an increased risk for hepatoblastoma),[50] radiation exposure, and prior treatment of cancer. Viral associations with cancer include EBV with malignant lymphomas, hepatitis B and C with hepatocellular carcinoma, and human immunodeficiency virus with lymphomas, Kaposi sarcoma, and other cancers.[51–53] Immunodeficiency, whether inherited or acquired, such as during posttransplant immune suppression therapy, predisposes to lymphomas and related lymphoproliferative disorders.[54,55] Treatment with chemotherapy, radiation therapy, and/or bone marrow transplant for a prior oncologic diagnosis also carries the risk of a secondary malignancy. In school-aged children with prior exposure to topoisomerase II inhibitors, anthracyclines, or alkylating agents, secondary AML may develop as a consequence of the DNA damage associated with these medications.[56]

ONCOLOGIC EMERGENCIES

There are times when it is not appropriate to initiate a thorough work-up for a malignancy as an outpatient. If a patient presents with the following problems they need immediate referral to a tertiary care center: vital sign instability, spinal cord compression, hyperleukocytosis (white blood cell [WBC] count >100,000 cells/ μL), tumor lysis syndrome (ie, increased uric acid level, hyperkalemia, acute renal failure, hyperphosphatemia), superior vena cava syndrome, hydrocephalus, neurologic instability (eg, seizure, altered mental status), cardiac tamponade, mediastinal mass, and/or respiratory compromise. These presentations of cancer are life threatening and need to be stabilized before a more complete work-up.

SUMMARY

Because of the rarity of cancer in the pediatric patient population, diagnosis is often delayed.[3,47] It is important for primary care physicians to have a high level of suspicion in patients who present with uncommon symptoms or persistence of symptoms despite appropriate interventions. Close follow-up and early referral to a pediatric oncologist are essential in the diagnosis of pediatric cancer.

REFERENCES

1. Pizzo PA, Poplack DG. Principles and practice of pediatric oncology. 6th edition. Philadelphia: Wolters Kluwer/Lippincott Williams & Wilkins Health; 2011.
2. Ahrensberg JM, Olesen F, Hansen RP, et al. Childhood cancer and factors related to prolonged diagnostic intervals: a Danish population-based study. Br J Cancer 2013;108(6):1280–7.
3. Haimi M, Peretz Nahum M, Ben Arush MW. Delay in diagnosis of children with cancer: a retrospective study of 315 children. Pediatr Hematol Oncol 2004; 21(1):37–48.
4. Young G, Toretsky JA, Campbell AB, et al. Recognition of common childhood malignancies. Am Fam Physician 2000;61(7):2144–54.
5. Gatta G, Botta L, Rossi S, et al. Childhood cancer survival in Europe 1999-2007: results of EUROCARE-5–a population-based study. Lancet Oncol 2014;15(1):35–47.
6. Raab CP, Gartner JC Jr. Diagnosis of childhood cancer. Prim Care 2009;36(4): 671–84.
7. Ward E, Desantis C, Robbins A, et al. Childhood and adolescent cancer statistics, 2014. CA Cancer J Clin 2014;64(2):83–103.
8. Jonsson OG, Sartain P, Ducore JM, et al. Bone pain as an initial symptom of childhood acute lymphoblastic leukemia: association with nearly normal hematologic indexes. J Pediatr 1990;117(2 Pt 1):233–7.
9. Bernbeck B, Wuller D, Janssen G, et al. Symptoms of childhood acute lymphoblastic leukemia: red flags to recognize leukemia in daily practice. Klin Padiatr 2009;221(6):369–73.
10. Friedmann AM. Evaluation and management of lymphadenopathy in children. Pediatr Rev 2008;29(2):53–60.

11. Herzog LW. Prevalence of lymphadenopathy of the head and neck in infants and children. Clin Pediatr (Phila) 1983;22(7):485–7.
12. Alam K, Khan R, Jain A, et al. The value of fine-needle aspiration cytology in the evaluation of pediatric head and neck tumors. Int J Pediatr Otorhinolaryngol 2009;73(7):923–7.
13. Siegel R, Naishadham D, Jemal A. Cancer statistics, 2013. CA Cancer J Clin 2013;63(1):11–30.
14. Dolecek TA, Propp JM, Stroup NE, et al. CBTRUS statistical report: primary brain and central nervous system tumors diagnosed in the United States in 2005-2009. Neuro Oncol 2012;14(Suppl 5):v1–49.
15. Patel S, Bhatnagar A, Wear C, et al. Are pediatric brain tumors on the rise in the USA? Significant incidence and survival findings from the SEER database analysis. Childs Nerv Syst 2014;30(1):147–54.
16. Sethi RV, Marino R, Niemierko A, et al. Delayed diagnosis in children with intracranial germ cell tumors. J Pediatr 2013;163(5):1448–53.
17. Phi JH, Kim SK, Lee YA, et al. Latency of intracranial germ cell tumors and diagnosis delay. Childs Nerv Syst 2013;29(10):1871–81.
18. Lanphear J, Sarnaik S. Presenting symptoms of pediatric brain tumors diagnosed in the emergency department. Pediatr Emerg Care 2014;30(2):77–80.
19. Wilne S, Collier J, Kennedy C, et al. Presentation of childhood CNS tumours: a systematic review and meta-analysis. Lancet Oncol 2007;8(8):685–95.
20. Ho CH, Chen SJ, Juan CJ, et al. Sudden death due to medulloblastoma: a case report. Acta Neurol Taiwan 2013;22(2):76–80.
21. Shemie S, Jay V, Rutka J, et al. Acute obstructive hydrocephalus and sudden death in children. Ann Emerg Med 1997;29(4):524–8.
22. Sandyk R. Acute deterioration and death in infancy due to posterior fossa tumour. A case report. S Afr Med J 1981;60(6):253–4.
23. Hsu W, Jallo GI. Pediatric spinal tumors. Handb Clin Neurol 2013;112:959–65.
24. Gross BA, Smith ER, Scott RM. Cavernous malformations of the basal ganglia in children. Journal of neurosurgery. Pediatrics 2013;12(2):171–4.
25. Saleh M, Carter MT, Latino GA, et al. Brain arteriovenous malformations in patients with hereditary hemorrhagic telangiectasia: clinical presentation and anatomical distribution. Pediatr Neurol 2013;49(6):445–50.
26. Fellah S, Callot V, Viout P, et al. Epileptogenic brain lesions in children: the added-value of combined diffusion imaging and proton MR spectroscopy to the pre-surgical differential diagnosis. Childs Nerv Syst 2012;28(2):273–82.
27. Gupta DK, Suri A, Mahapatra AK, et al. Intracranial Rosai-Dorfman disease in a child mimicking bilateral giant petroclival meningiomas: a case report and review of literature. Childs Nerv Syst 2006;22(9):1194–200.
28. Marchand I, Barkaoui MA, Garel C, et al. Central diabetes insipidus as the inaugural manifestation of Langerhans cell histiocytosis: natural history and medical evaluation of 26 children and adolescents. J Clin Endocrinol Metab 2011;96(9):E1352–60.
29. Wilne S, Walker D. Spine and spinal cord tumours in children: a diagnostic and therapeutic challenge to healthcare systems. Arch Dis Child Educ Pract Ed 2010;95(2):47–54.
30. Varan A, Atas E, Aydin B, et al. Evaluation of patients with intracranial tumors and central diabetes insipidus. Pediatr Hematol Oncol 2013;30(7):668–73.
31. Mazloom A, Zangeneh AH, Paulino AC. Prognostic factors after extraneural metastasis of medulloblastoma. Int J Radiat Oncol Biol Phys 2010;78(1):72–8.
32. Echevarria ME, Fangusaro J, Goldman S. Pediatric central nervous system germ cell tumors: a review. Oncologist 2008;13(6):690–9.

33. Park JR, Eggert A, Caron H. Neuroblastoma: biology, prognosis, and treatment. Pediatr Clin North Am 2008;55(1):97–120, x.
34. Weinstein JL, Katzenstein HM, Cohn SL. Advances in the diagnosis and treatment of neuroblastoma. Oncologist 2003;8(3):278–92.
35. Castleberry RP. Biology and treatment of neuroblastoma. Pediatr Clin North Am 1997;44(4):919–37.
36. Schilling FH, Spix C, Berthold F, et al. Neuroblastoma screening at one year of age. N Engl J Med 2002;346(14):1047–53.
37. Woods WG, Gao RN, Shuster JJ, et al. Screening of infants and mortality due to neuroblastoma. N Engl J Med 2002;346(14):1041–6.
38. Maris JM. Recent advances in neuroblastoma. N Engl J Med 2010;362(23): 2202–11.
39. Neville HL, Ritchey ML. Wilms' tumor. Overview of National Wilms' Tumor Study Group results. Urol Clin North Am 2000;27(3):435–42.
40. Kaste SC, Dome JS, Babyn PS, et al. Wilms tumour: prognostic factors, staging, therapy and late effects. Pediatr Radiol 2008;38(1):2–17.
41. Miller RW, Fraumeni JF Jr, Manning MD. Association of Wilms's tumor with aniridia, hemihypertrophy and other congenital malformations. N Engl J Med 1964; 270:922–7.
42. Fraumeni JF Jr, Geiser CF, Manning MD. Wilms' tumor and congenital hemihypertrophy: report of five new cases and review of literature. Pediatrics 1967;40(5): 886–99.
43. Scott RH, Stiller CA, Walker L, et al. Syndromes and constitutional chromosomal abnormalities associated with Wilms tumour. J Med Genet 2006;43(9):705–15.
44. D'Angio GJ. Pre- or postoperative therapy for Wilms' tumor? J Clin Oncol 2008; 26(25):4055–7.
45. Lemerle J, Voute PA, Tournade MF, et al. Preoperative versus postoperative radiotherapy, single versus multiple courses of actinomycin D, in the treatment of Wilms' tumor. Preliminary results of a controlled clinical trial conducted by the International Society of Paediatric Oncology (S.I.O.P.). Cancer 1976;38(2):647–54.
46. Newton WA Jr, Meadows AT, Shimada H, et al. Bone sarcomas as second malignant neoplasms following childhood cancer. Cancer 1991;67(1):193–201.
47. Haimi M, Perez-Nahum M, Stein N, et al. The role of the doctor and the medical system in the diagnostic delay in pediatric malignancies. Cancer Epidemiol 2011; 35(1):83–9.
48. Grimer RJ. Size matters for sarcomas! Ann R Coll Surg Engl 2006;88(6):519–24.
49. Grimer R, Athanasou N, Gerrand C, et al. UK guidelines for the management of bone sarcomas. Sarcoma 2010;2010:317462.
50. Heck JE, Meyers TJ, Lombardi C, et al. Case-control study of birth characteristics and the risk of hepatoblastoma. Cancer Epidemiol 2013;37(4):390–5.
51. Kanegane H, Nomura K, Miyawaki T, et al. Biological aspects of Epstein-Barr virus (EBV)-infected lymphocytes in chronic active EBV infection and associated malignancies. Crit Rev Oncol Hematol 2002;44(3):239–49.
52. Wen WH, Chang MH, Hsu HY, et al. The development of hepatocellular carcinoma among prospectively followed children with chronic hepatitis B virus infection. J Pediatr 2004;144(3):397–9.
53. McClain KL, Joshi VV, Murphy SB. Cancers in children with HIV infection. Hematol Oncol Clin North Am 1996;10(5):1189–201.
54. Rezaei N, Hedayat M, Aghamohammadi A, et al. Primary immunodeficiency diseases associated with increased susceptibility to viral infections and malignancies. J Allergy Clin Immunol 2011;127(6):1329–41.e2 [quiz: 1342–3].

55. Buell JF, Gross TG, Thomas MJ, et al. Malignancy in pediatric transplant recipients. Semin Pediatr Surg 2006;15(3):179–87.
56. Hijiya N, Ness KK, Ribeiro RC, et al. Acute leukemia as a secondary malignancy in children and adolescents: current findings and issues. Cancer 2009;115(1): 23–35.

Sudden Cardiac Death in Adolescents

Stefanie R. Ellison, MD

KEYWORDS

- Sudden death • Cardiac death • Electrical cardiac abnormalities
- Postoperative cardiac abnormalities • Syncope • Long QT syndrome
- Cardiomyopathy • Adolescent death

KEY POINTS

- Hypertrophic cardiomyopathy is the most common case of sudden cardiac death in adolescents.
- A detailed comprehensive history and physical examination, with a detailed family history and social history, are essential before participation in sports.
- The most common chief complaint of patients with sudden cardiac arrest is fatigue, near-syncope/lightheadedness, chest pain and then palpitations, in decreasing order of frequency.
- Seizures or seizure-like activity of ventricular tachycardia or ventricular fibrillation may distract physicians from considering these as warning signs of sudden cardiac death.

INTRODUCTION
Incidence

Sudden cardiac death (SCD) is defined as an abrupt, unexpected death resulting from a cardiovascular cause. Sudden is generally defined as death that occurs within 1 hour of the onset of symptoms, but can also occur within minutes for adolescents and children. The true incidence of adolescent SCD is unknown. Studies have determined the incidence to be 0.8 to 6.2 cases per 100,000 population per year.[1–6] Resuscitation that restores spontaneous circulation defines aborted sudden death. Actual resuscitated adolescent SCD data are even more difficult to obtain because databases are inaccurate and based on diagnosis and diagnostic codes. The US Centers for Disease Control and Prevention has estimated that 2000 patients 25 years of age and younger die from SCD each year.[7] Current studies have also demonstrated that the incidence of SCD in children and adolescents is on the rise.[8–10] In fact, SCD occurs more often in children and adolescents than infants because athletic participation increases the risk of SCD for those with underlying cardiovascular disease. Up to 25% of these deaths occur during sports.[11]

Department of Emergency Medicine, Truman Medical Center, University of Missouri-Kansas City, 2411 Holmes Street, Kansas City, MO 64108-2792, USA
E-mail address: ellisonst@umkc.edu

Prim Care Clin Office Pract 42 (2015) 57–76
http://dx.doi.org/10.1016/j.pop.2014.09.012   **primarycare.theclinics.com**

A study of high school and college athletes in the United States demonstrated that SCD occurs in fewer than 1 in 100,000 students.[11,12] Studies have further shown that sports participation in adolescents and young adults is attributable to underlying cardiac disorders compared with age-related, nonathletic populations.[12] More than 50% of athletic deaths owing to SCD occur in black athletes. It is also more common in young male athletes, occurring in a ratio of 1 to 9.[13] This may be in part that the most common sports with the occurrence of SCD are football and basketball and female participation in football differs greatly from that of the male gender.[13–15]

Patient Evaluation Overview and Pathophysiology

The known underlying cardiac disorders associated with adolescent SCD (**Box 1**) can be broken down into 3 categories: (1) Structural/functional, (2) primary electrical

---

Box 1
Cardiac disorders predisposing adolescents to sudden cardiac death

Structural/functional (in decreasing order of frequency)

Hypertrophic cardiomyopathy[a]

Coronary artery abnormalities

Myocarditis

Arrhythmogenic channelopathies/right ventricular cardiomyopathy[a]

Aortic rupture/Marfan syndrome[a]

Pulmonary hypertension

Dilated cardiomyopathy or restrictive cardiomyopathy[a]

Left ventricular outflow tract obstruction

Postoperative congenital heart disease[b]

Primary electrical abnormalities

Long QT syndrome[a]: Romano Ward, Jervell Lange Nielsen, Acquired

Brugada syndrome[a]

Wolff-Parkinson–White syndrome

Primary or idiopathic ventricular tachycardia/fibrillation

Catecholamine-exercise ventricular tachycardia[a]

Heart block-congenital, acquired

Short QT syndrome[a]

Acquired

Commotio cordis

Drugs of abuse—cocaine, stimulants, inhalants, gasoline, glue, nitrites, emetine

Primary pulmonary hypertension[a]

Secondary pulmonary hypertension

Atherosclerotic coronary artery disease

  [a] Familial/genetic.
  [b] Postoperative congenital heart diseases include tetralogy of Fallot, transposition with transportation of the great arteries, Fontan operation, hypoplastic left heart syndrome, coarctation of the aorta, cardiac transplantation.

abnormalities, and (3) acquired. **Fig. 1** provides a distribution of the most common cardiac causes of SCD in adolescent athletes.

CARDIAC DISORDERS PREDISPOSING ADOLESCENTS TO SUDDEN CARDIAC DEATH

This section focuses on the most common causes and mechanisms of SCD.

Hypertrophic Cardiomyopathy

Hypertrophic cardiomyopathy (HCM) affects more than 500,000 people in the United States and is the most common cause of SCD in adolescents.[14,16] Children under 12 make up less than 10% of all patients who have this disorder. The Pediatric Cardiomyopathy Registry reports that HCM occurs at a rate of 5 per 1 million children. HCM is among the most common inherited cardiac disorders affecting around 1 in 500 people and is the number 1 cause of SCD in young athletes.[13–16] It is a heterogeneous disorder, produced by mutations in multiple genes coding for sarcomeric proteins. Inheritance is primarily autosomal dominant, with variable penetrance. The annual mortality owing to HCM is estimated at around 1% to 2 %.[16]

HCM occurs when the muscle fibers of the heart are thickened and do not allow the heart to relax sufficiently for the heart to fill (**Fig. 2**). With the combination of poor filling and contractility owing to the stiff nature of the thickened muscles, the patient's heart may not pump adequate blood, especially during exercise. Any of the chambers can become hypertrophic, but it occurs more frequently in the left ventricle. HCM is also characterized by asymmetric septal hypertrophy with a disarray of ventricular muscle fibers, adding to the risk of arrhythmias, even in patients without hypertrophy. It should

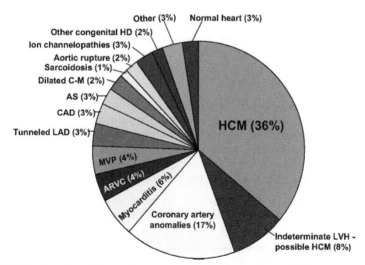

Fig. 1. Distribution of cardiovascular causes of sudden death in 1435 young competitive athletes. From the Minneapolis Heart Institute Foundation Registry, 1980 to 2005. ARVC, arrhythmogenic right ventricular cardiomyopathy; AS, aortic stenosis; CAD, coronary artery disease; C-M, cardiomyopathy; HD, heart disease; LAD, left anterior descending; LVH, left ventricular hypertrophy; MVP, mitral valve prolapse. (*From* Maron BJ, Thompson PD, Ackerman MJ, et al. Recommendations and considerations related to preparticipation screening for cardiovascular abnormalities in competitive athletes: 2007 update: a scientific statement from the American Heart Association Council on Nutrition, Physical Activity, and Metabolism: endorsed by the American College of Cardiology Foundation. Circulation 2007;115:1645; with permission.)

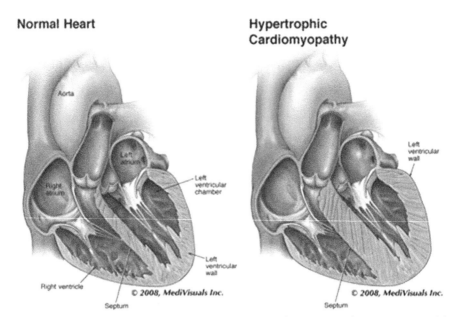

Normal Heart

Hypertrophic
Cardiomyopathy

Fig. 2. Normal heart versus hypertrophic cardiomyopathy anatomy. (*From* Barnes-Jewish Hospital. Hypertrophic Cardiomyopathy. Available at: http://www.barnesjewish.org/heart-vascular/hypertrophic-cardiomyopathy. Accessed March 10, 2014.)

also be noted that patients with HCM can have normal chest x-rays because the thickening may only occur in the septum. When the thickening includes the septum of the left ventricular outflow tract, then obstruction during systole can lead to hypertrophic obstructive cardiomyopathy. Only 25% of patients with HCM actually develop hypertrophic obstructive cardiomyopathy.[16,17]

The hypertrophic cardiomyopathy electrocardiogram

The chief abnormality associated with HCM is left ventricular hypertrophy and the degree and distribution of left ventricular hypertrophy is variable ranging from mild (13–15 mm) to severe myocardial thickening (30–60 mm).[18] The most commonly observed pattern comes from the asymmetrical thickening of the anterior interventricular septum. See **Fig. 3** for electrocardiographic (ECG) features.

Diagnostic electrocardiographic criteria for hypertrophic cardiomyopathy
- Left ventricular hypertrophy is shown by increased precordial voltages and nonspecific ST segment and T-wave changes.
- Asymmetrical septal hypertrophy produces deep, narrow "dagger-like" Q waves in the lateral (V5-6, I, aVL) and inferior (II, III, aVF) leads. Lateral Q waves are more common than inferior Q waves in HCM compared with prior myocardial infarction.
- Left atrial enlargement, or "P mitrale", on the ECG.

For 2 additional ECG demonstrations on patients with HCM, please view the following YouTube links detailing the diagnostic criteria by Professor Sanjay Sharma, Consultant Cardiologist in the CYR Center for Inherited Cardiac Diseases:

http://www.youtube.com/watch?v=pEHAotWgePY
http://www.youtube.com/watch?v=RULjhr4SEjs#t=68

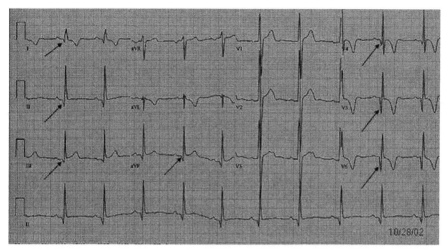

Fig. 3. Asymmetrical septal hypertrophy produces "dagger-like Q waves" in the lateral and inferior leads. (*From* Life in the Fast Lane. Hypertrophic Cardiomyopathy (HCM). Available at: http://lifeinthefastlane.com/ecg-library/hcm/. Life in the Fast Lane is licensed under a Creative Commons ShareAlike 4.0 International User's License http://creativecommons.org/licenses/by-sa/4.0/.)

Apical hypertrophic cardiomyopathy electrocardiogram

Apical HCM is less common but still important to diagnose in the screening of athletes.[17,18] There is localized hypertrophy in the left ventricular apex with classic ECG finding as demonstrated in **Fig. 4**.

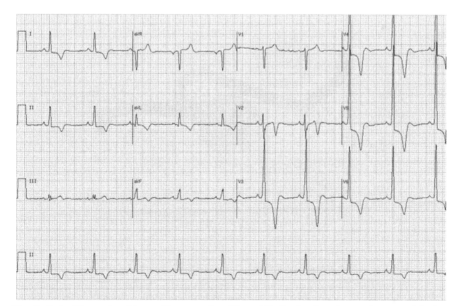

Fig. 4. Apical hypertrophic cardiomyopathy. (*From* Life in the Fast Lane. Hypertrophic Cardiomyopathy (HCM). Available at: http://lifeinthefastlane.com/ecg-library/hcm/. Life in the Fast Lane is licensed under a Creative Commons ShareAlike 4.0 International User's License http://creativecommons.org/licenses/by-sa/4.0/.)

Diagnostic electrocardiographic criteria for Apical Hypertrophic Cardiomyopathy
- High precordial voltages.
- Giant T-wave inversions in the precordial and high lateral leads.

There is an excellent video of a case report of HCM by Amal Mattu of a patient who presented with syncope: http://www.youtube.com/watch?v=RsNkhr4lhhU.

Coronary Artery Anomalies

Coronary artery anomalies are the second most common cause of SCD in adolescents in the United States.[19] The anomaly most often associated with SCD is the left coronary artery originating from the right sinus of Valsalva.[19–21] The artery then traverses between the aorta and pulmonary artery and when a patient exercises, the great vessels both increase in size and compress the left main coronary artery, causing ischemia (**Fig. 5**). These are difficult to identify with routine echocardiograms and can require imaging studies or angiography to diagnose. Symptoms include early fatigue, angina, or exercise-induced syncope and should direct the clinician to refer the patient for consultation and further studies.

Primary electrical abnormalities

There are a variety of primary arrhythmias that are a rare cause of SCD in young patients. These include the arrhythmic channelopathies and primary arrhythmias that can be determined by ECG. These cases of SCD are often preceded by recurrent syncope, which can trigger the workup before the arrhythmia gets more malignant. **Fig. 6** and **Table 1** pair the primary arrhythmia, the features, an example of the diagnostic ECG, and the treatment for long QT syndrome (LQTS), Brugada syndrome,

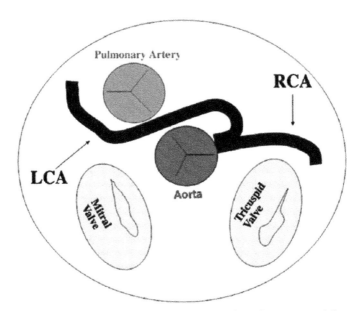

Fig. 5. Left coronary anomaly originating in the contralateral sinus. LCA, left coronary artery; RCA, right coronary artery. (*From* Barriales-Villa R, Morís de la Tassa C. Anomalías congénitas de las arterias coronarias con origen en el seno de Valsalva contralateral: ¿qué actitud se debe seguir? [Congenital coronary artery anomalies with origin in the contralateral sinus of Valsalva: which approach should we take?]. Rev Esp Cardiol 2006;59(4):365 [in Spanish]; with permission.)

A

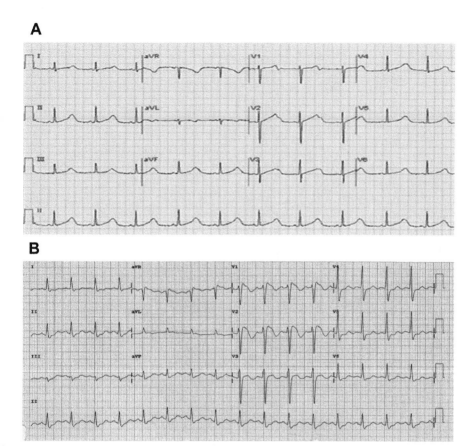

B

Fig. 6. Electrocardiographs of primary electrical abnormalities. (A) Long QT syndrome. (B) Brugada syndrome. (C) Wolff–Parkinson–White syndrome. (D) Dilated cardiomyopathy ventricular tachycardia/fibrillation. (E) Catecholamine–exercise ventricular tachycardia. (From [A] Image reprinted with permission from Medscape Reference (http://emedicine.medscape.com/), 2014, available at: http://reference.medscape.com/features/slideshow/syncope; and [B,E] From Life in the Fast Lane. Dilated Cardiomyopathy. Available at: http://lifeinthefastlane.com/ecg-library/dilated-cardiomyopathy/. Life in the Fast Lane is licensed under a Creative Commons ShareAlike 4.0 International User's License http://creativecommons.org/licenses/by-sa/4.0.)

Wolff–Parkinson–White syndrome, and dilated cardiomyopathy, ventricular tachycardia, and catecholamine exercise ventricular tachycardia.[22–26]

Long QT syndrome
LQTS is a genetic disorder that occurs in 1 in 2500 to 3000 individuals.[25] At least 10 genes have been associated with LQTS. Mutations in the genes responsible for potassium, sodium, and calcium channels in cardiac muscle have all been implicated in congenital LQTS. Congenital forms of LQTS include Romano–Ward, Jervell–Lange–Nielsen, Andersen, and Timothy syndromes. These are a variety of genetic abnormalities in the ion channels that make up an estimated 80% of patients with LQTS.[26,27] Many patients with LQTS have a QTc that is within the normal range, making the diagnosis difficult.[28] Obtaining a history of syncope, a family history of LQTS, or SCD should prompt the clinician to obtain an ECG. It is also helpful to know the medications that cause QT prolongation and put these patients at risk for arrhythmias (**Box 2**).

C

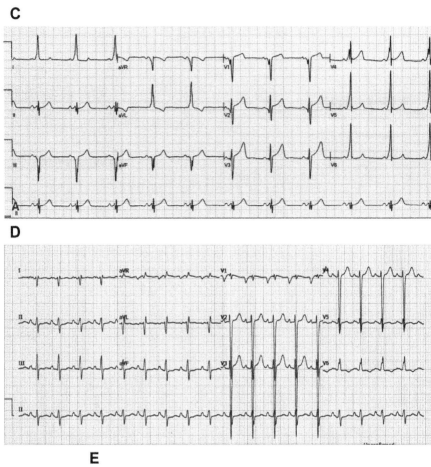

D

E

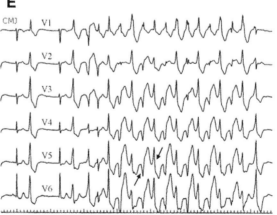

Fig. 6. (*continued*)

Table 1
Primary electrical abnormalities: features, electrocardiogram, and treatment

Primary Electrical Abnormalities	Features	ECG	Treatment
LQTS[22–24]: Romano Ward, Jervell Lange Nielsen, acquired	Familial genetic disorder Ion channel mutations Presents in Torsades de pointes Romano Ward is MC inherited LQTS Jervell-Lange has congenital deafness	See **Fig. 6A** [21]Prolonged QT measures from the onset of the Q wave to the end of the T wave in Lead II Varies with heart rate but >0.44 in men, >0.46 in children and women for HR 50–90/min is prolonged Torsades de pointes can occur Can deteriorate from polymorphic ventricular tachycardia to ventricular fibrillation	β-Blocker therapy Recommendations on exercise intensity by a cardiologist ICD if β-blockers fail
Brugada[25] syndrome	Inherited autosomal dominant arrhythmogenic syndrome characterized by life-threatening ventricular arrhythmias Genetic mutations are the cause	See **Fig. 6B** ECG abnormalities are from repolarization and depolarization abnormalities ST segment coved elevations in the right precordial leads J wave amplitude ≥2 mm followed by a negative T-wave	Placement of ICD
Wolff-Parkinson-White[26]	Owing to ≥1 more reentrant pathways inducing SVT or atrial fibrillation Up to 14% associated with malignant tachycardias Malignant arrhythmias from short reentrant pathway repolarization or multiple pathways	See **Fig. 6C** Short PR interval Delta waves present	Undergo EPT and ablation
Dilated cardiomyopathy ventricular tachycardia/fibrillation[27]	Cardiac dilation and systolic dysfunction Inherited or acquired Lamin AC gene mutations a common cause of DCM and SCD	See **Fig. 6D** Marked LVH Poor R wave progression Left atrial enlargement Right axis deviation	Permanent pacemaker and ICD placement
Catecholamine-exercise ventricular tachycardia[28]	Ventricular ectopy induced by exercise or emotional stress Mutation in gene that encodes Ca-mediated sarcoplasmic fibers Lethal in 30%–50% if left untreated	Pre-exercise ECG is usually normal, stress testing recommended ECG with exercise (see **Fig. 6E**) Nonsustained wide ventricular tachycardia	β-Blocker therapy Recommendations on exercise intensity by a cardiologist ICD if β-blockers fail

Abbreviations: DCM, dilated cardiomyopathy; ECG, electrocardiograph; EPT, electrophysiologic testing; HR, heart rate; ICD, implantable cardioverter defibrillator; LQTS, long QT syndrome; LVH, left ventricular hypertrophy; MC, most common; SCD, sudden cardiac death; SVT, supraventricular tachycardia.

Box 2
Examples of commonly used medications that cause acquired QT prolongation

Antiarrhythmics

Amiodarone (Cordarone)

Disopyramide (Norpace)

Dofetilide (Tikosyn)

Ibutilide (Corvert)

Procainamide (Pronestyl)

Quinidine (Quinaglute)

Sotalol (Betapace)

Antipsychotics

Chlorpromazine (Thorazine)

Clozapine (Clozaril)

Haloperidol (Haldol)

Quetiapine (Seroquel)

Risperidone (Risperdal)

Thioridazine (Mellaril)

Antibiotics

Azithromycin (Zithromax)

Ciprofloxacin (Cipro)

Clarithromycin (Biaxin)

Erythromycin (Erythrocin)

Fluconazole (Diflucan)

Gatifloxacin (Tequin)

Itraconazole (Sporanox)

Ketoconazole (Nizoral)

Levofloxacin (Levaquin)

Moxifloxacin (Avelox)

Ofloxacin (Floxin)

Sparfloxacin (Zagam)

Telithromycin (Ketek)

Trimethoprim-Sulfa (Bactrim)

Antidepressants

Amitriptyline (Elavil)

Citalopram (Celexa)

Desipramine (Pertofrane)

Doxepin (Sinequan)

Fluoxetine (Prozac)

Imipramine (Norfranil)

Nortriptyline (Pamelor)

Paroxetine (Paxil)

Sertraline (Zoloft)

Venlafaxine (Effexor)

Antiemetics

Ondansetron (Zofran)

Prochlorperazine (Compazine)

Data from Ayad R, Assar M, Simpson L, et al. Causes and management of drug-induced long QT syndrome. Proc (Bayl Univ Med Cent) 2010;23(3):250–5.

Congenital Heart Disease Risk

The incidence of sudden death in patients with congenital heart disease is about 100 in 100,000 patient-years, owing to arrhythmic, embolic, or circulatory causes.[29] Specifically, tetralogy of Fallot is associated with higher incidence rates of known ventricular tachycardia and intra-atrial re-entrant tachycardia and a 0.5% to 6% risk of SCD.[30] Patients who are status post Fontan procedure also have high acquired arrhythmia rates with an increased incidence of SCD.

DIAGNOSIS AND SCREENING: PREPARTICIPATION HISTORY AND PHYSICAL EXAMINATION

A detailed comprehensive history and physical examination, with a detailed family history and social history are essential before participation in sports. Although state laws vary, the law generally requires that before students may participate in organized sports that individual physicians must use reasonable care in detecting and identifying medical abnormalities that may cause sudden death or serious injury.[31] It is important to screen for a history of near syncope, syncope, chest pain, palpitations, lightheadedness, and shortness of breath. It is also important to establish a clear and detailed history of SCD in relatives, premature placement of pacemakers, or internal cardiac defibrillators to adequately inquire about the risk to your patient. Questionnaires and electronic medical records may assist this detailed history and guide the primary care physicians or pediatricians to identify undiagnosed patients with SCD risk. There is a 3-generation pedigree family history tool available from the US Surgeon General's Family History Initiative at www.hhs.gov/familyhistory.

Warning Signs and Symptoms

Symptoms of dizziness, lightheadedness, chest pain, syncope, palpitations, dyspnea, and a family history of SCD were noted in 25% to 61% of the population studied. Deaths were exercise or exertion related in 8% to 33% of the SCD cases.[32,33] In 1 study, patients complained most often of recent fatigue (44%), followed by near syncope or lightheadednesss (30%), chest pain or palpitations (28%), shortness of breath (23%), syncope (18%), or unexplained seizure (23%).[33] Seizures or seizurelike activity of ventricular tachycardia or ventricular fibrillation may distract physicians from considering these warning signs of SCD. Neurologic signs and symptoms may direct primary physicians to refer to neurology over making the appropriate referral to cardiology. Episodes of syncope or presyncope are the most common presenting signs of lethal ventricular tachyarrhythmias. Coronary artery abnormalities or aortic dissection present with chest pain. Cardiomyopathies that lead to pulmonary congestion or edema may present as "cardiac wheezing" and be misinterpreted as bronchospasm or reactive airway disease. To guide the physician, the American Heart Association offers a 12-element screening tool for preparticipation screening of competitive athletes that is considered a complete set of questions (**Box 3**).[34]

Table 2 demonstrates the number of patients who had symptoms reported to their physicians and the timing before SCD. Of this cohort, preparticipation evaluations were completed in 61% of children an average of 15.6 months before SCD, and a well-child evaluations were completed in 60% of children an average of 12.6 months before SCD.[35]

Physical Examination

A detailed physical examination should always be paired with a thorough history and family history, even though it does not commonly yield positive findings. Screening is

---

Box 3

The 12-Element American Heart Association recommendations for preparticipation cardiovascular screening of competitive athletes

Medical history[a]

Personal history

1. Exertional chest pain/discomfort

2. Unexplained syncope/near syncope[b]

3. Excessive exertional and unexplained dyspnea/fatigue, associated with exercise

4. Prior recognition of a heart murmur

5. Elevated systemic blood pressure

Family history

6. Premature death (sudden and unexpected, or otherwise) before age 50 years owing to heart disease, in 1 or more relatives

7. Disability from heart disease in a close relative less than 50 years of age

8. Specific knowledge of certain cardiac conditions in family members: hypertrophic or dilated cardiomyopathy, long QT syndrome or other ion channelopathies, Marfan syndrome, or clinically important arrhythmias

Physical examination

9. Heart murmur[c]

10. Femoral pulses to exclude aortic coarctation

11. Physical stigmata of Marfan syndrome

12. Brachial artery blood pressure (sitting position)[d]

   [a] Parental verification is recommended for high school and middle school athletes.
   [b] Judged not to be neurocardiogenic (vasovagal); of particular concern when related to exertion.
   [c] Auscultation should be performed in both supine and standing positions (or with Valsalva maneuver), specifically to identify murmurs of dynamic left ventricular outflow tract obstruction.
   [d] Preferably taken in both arms.
   From Maron BJ, Thompson PD, Ackerman MJ, et al. Recommendations and considerations related to preparticipation screening for cardiovascular abnormalities in competitive athletes: 2007 update: a scientific statement from the American Heart Association Council on Nutrition, Physical Activity, and Metabolism: endorsed by the American College of Cardiology Foundation. Circulation 2007;115:1652; with permission.

Table 2
Reported Symptom Prevalence in Children and Young Adults with Sudden Cardiac Arrest (SCA)

Symptom	Study Population with Symptom (%)	SCA Victims with Symptoms Before Their Most Recent Physician Visit (%)	Symptom Onset Before SCA (mo)
Fatigue	44	25	21
Near-syncope/lightheadedness	30	22	30
Chest pain/discomfort	28	20	26
Palpitations	28	17	25
Heart murmur	24	—	89
Shortness of breath	23	20	19
Tire more easily than friends	22	—	NA
Syncope	18	14	47
Unexplained seizure activity	13	11	71
Decrease in physical activity	11	—	NA
Hypertension	3	—	25
One of the above symptoms	72	51	—

Timing of symptoms related to most recent physician visit and SCA is provided.
Abbreviation: NA, not applicable.
Adapted from Drezner J, Fudge J, Harman K, et al. Warning symptoms and family history in children and young adults with sudden cardiac arrest. J Am Board Fam Med 2012;23(4):408–15.

designed to identify or raise suspicion of cardiovascular abnormalities that could lead to sudden death. The key elements of the physical examination are as follows.

- Blood pressure measurement.
- A complete cardiovascular examination with attention to heart rate, regularity, murmur, gallop, or rub (the presence of a loud systolic heart murmur should create suspicion for congenital aortic valve stenosis).
- Peripheral circulation and palpation of all pulses may yield positive findings of coarctation of the aorta.
- Signs of Marfan syndrome and the inherent risk of aortic dissection. Refer to **Box 3** for the elements of the physical examination recommended by the American Heart Association.[34–37] **Box 4** further characterizes the signs and symptoms of structural causes of SCD.

ACQUIRED CAUSES
Commotio Cordis

Commotio cordis is a relatively rare cause of SCD that occurs most often in males under the age of 18. It is caused by a direct blow over the heart that is timed just before the T-wave peak during a vulnerable phase of repolarization.[38] Collapse occurs immediately or occurs after a brief period of lightheadedness. The rhythm disturbance is usually ventricular fibrillation. Survival rate is low at around 25% to 35% and only owing to bystander cardiopulmonary resuscitation and defibrillation.[38] Most reported cases are due to baseball, so chest protectors have been suggested as a preventative measure. Additionally, increased education on cardiopulmonary resuscitation and the use of automated external defibrillators for the community could also potentially decrease SCD from commotion cordis.[30]

Box 4
Signs and symptoms of underlying structural cardiac causes of sudden cardiac death (SCD)

Hypertrophic cardiomyopathy

Can be asymptomatic

Dyspnea

Angina

Presyncope

Syncope

Exercise intolerance or palpitations

Symptoms of heart failure

Hypertrophic obstructive cardiomyopathy: LV outflow tract obstruction

Chest pain

Palpitations

Syncope

Signs of LV heart failure

Arrhythmogenic right ventricular cardiomyopathy

Palpitations

Lightheadedness

Chest pain

Syncope

Signs of heart failure (rare): Shortness of breath, swelling of the feet and ankles, fatigue

Aortic rupture/Marfan syndrome

A tall, thin build

Long arms, legs, fingers, and toes and flexible joints

Scoliosis

Pectus excavatum and pectus carinatum

Teeth that are overcrowded

Flat feet

Micrognathia

Coronary artery abnormalities

Early fatigue

Chest pain or angina

Atypical chest pain and/or syncope that occurs with exercise

Pulmonary hypertension

Dyspnea on exertion

Fatigue

Dizziness

Syncope

Myocarditis

Chest pain

Arrhythmia

Shortness of breath, at rest or during physical activity

Peripheral edema

Fatigue

Other signs and symptoms you would have with a viral infection, such as a headache, body aches, joint pain, fever, a sore throat or diarrhea

Dilated cardiomyopathy or restrictive cardiomyopathy

Fatigue and weakness

Dyspnea on exertion or orthopnea

Reduced ability to exercise

Lightheadedness, dizziness or syncope

Persistent cough or wheezing, especially when lying down

Edema

Ascites

Sudden weight gain

Anorexia

Palpitations

Pallor

Abbreviation: LV, left ventricular.
    Data from Refs.[37–39]

Drugs of Abuse

Performance-enhancing drugs have been linked to SCD in adolescent athletes. Illicit substances such as anabolic steroids, stimulants such as ephedra, and peptide hormones have been linked to a range of cardiac arrhythmias in healthy subjects.[39] Other drugs of abuse such as cocaine, heroin, marijuana, amphetamines, ecstasy, inhalants, gasoline, glue, and emetine have also been known to cause sudden death in users.[40]

Electrocardiogram, Echocardiogram, and Genetic Testing

Recent high-profile athlete deaths and the media have placed a greater emphasis on the need to screen athletes before participating in competitive athletics. The American College of Cardiology states that it is only necessary to provide preparticipation evaluation of athletes to detect possible cardiovascular abnormalities to prevent SCD.[34] The use of ECG in the routine testing of the preparticipation evaluation of athletes is not currently recommended by the American College of Cardiology and remains controversial. In 2004 and 2005, European investigators and the International Olympic Committee recommended the use of the 12-lead ECG as a strategy for screening athletes. ECGs are abnormal in more than 90% of patients with HCM and the ECG is effective at detecting LQTS and Brugada syndrome.[4] It should also be remembered that the resting ECG is abnormal owing to the changes in the trained athlete's heart. In addition, exercise-induced conduction abnormalities such as catecholaminergic ventricular tachycardia should undergo stress tests because the resting ECG can be normal.

Routine testing with ECG is recommended during the initial evaluation of any child or young adult with syncope. A cardiac cause for syncope was identified in 22 patients (5%), and was LQTS (n = 14), arrhythmias (n = 6), and cardiomyopathies (n = 2). An abnormal history, physical examination, or ECG identified 21 of the 22 patients with a cardiac cause of syncope (96% sensitivity; 99% negative predictive value).[41,42] If the history and physical examination are typical for neurocardiogenic syncope but the ECG is normal, further testing generally is not needed.

Echocardiogram

Syncope occurring during exercise is an especially ominous sign and warrants a high index of suspicion for underlying cardiac disease. If the preparticipation history and physical examination discovers exertional syncope, the diagnostic workup should be performed in consultation with a cardiologist. The workup should include an ECG, echocardiogram, stress ECG, and possibly advanced cardiac imaging to identify and rule out rare structural abnormalities such as arrhythmogenic right ventricular cardiomyopathy or congenital coronary artery anomalies. In a review of 474 athletes with a history of syncope or near syncope discovered during preparticipation screening, 33% with syncope that occurred during exercise were found to have a structural cardiac disease known to cause SCD.[43]

GENETIC CAUSES OF ADOLESCENT SUDDEN CARDIAC DEATH

As **Box 1** demonstrates, there are a significant number of familial and genetic conditions that are linked with SCD. There is increasing evidence of genetic mutations in seemingly normal and healthy individuals that are linked to SCD. Specifically, HCM and the cardiac channelopathies are now known to be genetic.[26-28] There are now studies that justify testing of genetic phenotyping of relatives that have died of SCD. Tester and Ackerman[27] reported 17 cases demonstrating genetic evidence for LQTS or for catacholaminergic polymorphic ventricular tachycardia mutations; 9 (53%) of these cases had a family history of SCD or syncope documented in the medical record. Genetic testing can also serve as a screening tool; testing of family members has revealed an additional 151 undiagnosed or asymptomatic disease carriers or 8.9 per family.[27,44] Postmortem genetic screening, or the "molecular autopsy," can also be an important method to identify the cause of SCD and to provide screening for at-risk family members. In postmortem genetic testing in cases of autopsy-negative sudden unexplained death, more than one third of cases were found to have a pathologic cardiac ion channel mutation.[45-48]

PREVENTION AND SCREENING PROGRAMS AND EDUCATION

There is proven benefit in the use of ECGs to screen athletes for cardiac abnormalities that put them at risk of SCD. There has been demonstrated success for screening in athletes in Italy, Israel, Japan, and the United States, so currently the American Heart Association and American Association of Pediatrics jointly endorse the use of ECGs in the initial screening of athletes. **Fig. 7** provides an example algorithm for Hypertrophic cardiomyopathy cardiac subspecialty evaluation and management. However, studies examining the cost effectiveness of screening programs for athletes that include an ECG in screening have demonstrated that they are generally unfavorable owing to the low prevalence and imperfect screening and diagnostic specificity. The cost placed on society reflects a high use of resources that leads to a large number of healthy children be referred for follow-up testing.[49]

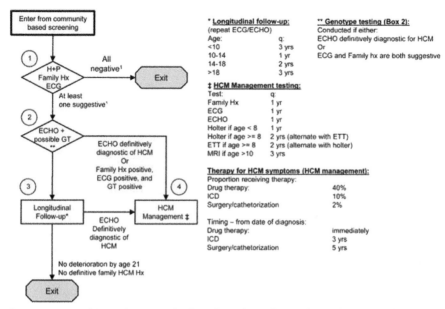

Fig. 7. Hypertrophic cardiomyopathy (HCM) cardiac subspecialty evaluation and management. ECG, electrocardiograph; ECHO, echocardiography; ETT, exercise tolerance test; H+P, history and physical examination; Hx, history; ICD, implantable cardioverter defibrillator. (*From* Leslie L, Cohen J, Newburger J, et al. Costs and benefits of targeted screening for causes of sudden cardiac death in children and adolescents. Circulation 2012;125(21):2626; with permission.)

SUMMARY

SCD in adolescents is devastating but potentially preventable. Consistent preparticipation screening by primary care physicians and pediatricians with a focus on a history of syncope, exertional chest pain, and a family history of SCD paired with a physical examination can guide the appropriate testing and referral for high-risk patients. The cost effectiveness of routine screening ECGs is still under debate. Treatment and monitoring for underlying cardiac disease can save lives and recommendations for decreased physical activity may also be necessary.

REFERENCES

1. Corrado D, Basso C, Pavei A, et al. Trends in sudden cardiovascular death in young competitive athletes after implementation of a preparticipation screening program. JAMA 2006;296:1593–601 CrossRefMedline.
2. Maron BJ, Doerer JJ, Haas TS, et al. Sudden deaths in young competitive athletes: analysis of 1866 deaths in the United States, 1980–2006. Circulation 2009;119:1085–92.
3. Corrado D, Basso C, Schiavon M, et al. Screening for hypertrophic cardiomyopathy in young athletes. N Engl J Med 1998;339(6):364–9.
4. Driscoll DJ, Edwards WD. Sudden unexpected death in children and adolescents. J Am Coll Cardiol 1985;5(Suppl 6):118B–21B.
5. Wren C. Sudden death in children and adolescents. Heart 2002;88(4):426–31.
6. Neuspiel DR, Kuller LH. Sudden and un-expected natural death in childhood and adolescence. JAMA 1985;254(10):1321–5.

7. Kung HC, Hoyert DL, Xu J, et al. Deaths: final data for 2005. Natl Vital Stat Rep 2008;56(10):1–120.
8. Shen WK, Edwards WD, Hammill SC, et al. Sudden un- expected nontraumatic death in 54 young adults: a 30-year population-based study. Am J Cardiol 1995;76(3):148–52.
9. SoRelle R. Jump in sudden deaths reported in younger people during past decade. Circulation 2001;103(10):e9019–21.
10. Spurgeon D. Sudden cardiac deaths rise 10% in young Americans. BMJ 2001; 322(7286):573.
11. O'Connor FG, Kugler JP, Oriscello RG. Sudden death in young athletes: screening for the needle in a haystack. Am Fam Physician 1998;57:2763–70.
12. Corrado D, Basso C, Rizzoli G, et al. Does sports activity enhance the risk of sudden death in adolescents and young adults? J Am Coll Cardiol 2003; 42(11):1959–63.
13. Maron BJ, Carney KP, Lever HM, et al. Relationship of race to sudden cardiac death in competitive athletes with hypertrophic cardiomyopathy. J Am Coll Cardiol 2003;41:974–80.
14. Maron BJ, Shirani J, Poliac LC, et al. Sudden death in young competitive athletes: clinical, demographic, and pathological profiles. JAMA 1996;276:199–204.
15. Van Camp SP, Bloor CM, Mueller FO, et al. Nontraumatic sports death in high school and college athletes. Med Sci Sports Exerc 1995;27:641–7.
16. Maron BJ. Hypertrophic cardiomyopathy. Lancet 1997;350(9071):127–33.
17. Kelly BS, Mattu A, Brady WJ. Hypertrophic cardiomyopathy: electrocardio-graphic manifestations and other important considerations for the emergency physician. Am J Emerg Med 2007;25(1):72–9.
18. Life in the Fastlane. Hypertrophic cardiomyopathy (HCM). Available at: http://lifeinthefastlane.com/ecg-library/hcm/. Accessed March 8, 2014.
19. Corrado D, Thiene G, Cocco P, et al. Non-atherosclerotic coronary artery disease and sudden death in the young. Br Heart J 1992;68:601–7.
20. Nakamura CT, Canete DR, Lau JM. A review of the anomalous origin of the left coronary artery from the anterior sinus of Valsalva: is prevention possible? Hawaii Med J 1993;52:294–9.
21. Lipsett J, Cohle SD, Berry PJ, et al. Anomalous coronary arteries: a multicenter pediatric autopsy study. Pediatr Pathol 1994;14:287–300.
22. Wilde A, Antzelevitch C, Borggrefe M, et al. Proposed Diagnostic cretieria for the Brugada Syndrome: consensus report. Circulation 2002;106:2514–9. http://dx.doi.org/10.1161/01.CIR.0000034169.45752.4A.
23. Pappone C, Vicedomini G, Manguso F, et al. Risk of malignant arrhythmias in initially symptomatic patients with Wolff-Parkinson-White syndrome: results of a prospective long-term electrophysiological follow-up study. Circulation 2012; 125:661–8.
24. Dadkhah S, Dowlatshahi S, Sharain K, et al. Exercise induced non-sustained ventricular tachycardia and indication for invasive management. Clin Med Insights Cardiol 2011;5:121–6.
25. Schwartz PJ, Stramba-Badiale M, Crotti L, et al. Prevalence of the congenital long-QT syndrome. Circulation 2009;120:1761–7.
26. Lehnart SE, Ackerman MJ, Benson DW Jr, et al. Inherited arrhythmias: a National Heart, Lung, and Blood Institute and Office of Rare Diseases workshop consensus report about the diagnosis, phenotyping, molecular mechanisms, and therapeutic approaches for primary cardiomyopathies of gene mutations affecting ion channel function. Circulation 2007;116(20):2325–45.

27. Tester DJ, Ackerman MJ. Postmortem long QT syndrome genetic testing for sudden unexplained death in the young. J Am Coll Cardiol 2007;49(2):240–6.

28. Vincent GM, Timothy KW, Leppert M, et al. The spectrum of symptoms and QT intervals in carriers of the gene for the long-QT syndrome. New Engl J Med 1992;327:846–52.

29. Silka MJ, Hardy BG, Menashe VD, et al. A population-based prospective evaluation of risk of sudden cardiac death after operation for common congenital heart defects. J Am Coll Cardiol 1998;32:245–51.

30. Gajewski K, Saul J. Sudden cardiac death in children and adolescents (excluding Sudden Infant Death Syndrome). Ann Pediatr Cardiol 2010;3(2): 107–12.

31. Mitton MI. Emerging legal issues in sports medicine. St John's L Rev 2002;76:5–86. Available at: http://scholarship.law.stjohns.edu/lawreview/vol76/iss1/2. Accessed March 2014.

32. Liberthson RR. Sudden death from cardiac causes in children and young adults. N Engl J Med 1996;334(16):1039–44.

33. Wisten A, Messner T. Symptoms preceding sudden cardiac death in the young are common but often misinterpreted. Scand Cardiovasc J 2005;39(3):143–9.

34. Maron BJ, Thompson PD, Ackerman MJ, et al. Recommendations and considerations related to preparticipation screening for cardiovascular abnormalities in competitive athletes: 2007 update: a scientific statement from the American Heart Association Council on Nutrition, Physical Activity, and Metabolism: endorsed by the American College of Cardiology Foundation. Circulation 2007;115:1643–55.

35. Drezner J, Fudge J, Harman K, et al. Warning symptoms and family history in children and young adults with sudden cardiac arrest. J Am Board Fam Med 2012;23(4):408–15.

36. Pelliccia A. Congenital coronary artery anomalies in young patients. New perspectives for timely identification. J Am Coll Cardiol 2001;37(2):598–600.

37. Maron BJ, Douglas PS, Graham TP, et al. Task Force 1: preparticipation screening and diagnosis of cardiovascular disease in athletes. J Am Coll Cardiol 2005;45:1322–6.

38. Link MS, Wang PJ, Pandian NG, et al. An experimental model of sudden death due to low-energy chest-wall impact (commotio cordis). N Engl J Med 1998; 338:1805–11.

39. Furlanello F, Bentivegna S, Cappato R, et al. Arrhythmogenic effects of illicit drugs in athletes. Ital Heart J 2003;4(12):829–37.

40. Montagnana M, Lippi G, Franchini M, et al. Sudden cardiac death in young athletes. Intern Med 2008;47:1–20.

41. Maron BJ, Mckenna WJ, Danielson GK. American College of Cardiology/European Society of Cardiology clinical expert consensus document on hypertrophic cardiomyopathy. A report of the American College of Cardiology Foundation Task Force on Clinical Expert Consensus Documents and the European Society of Cardiology Committee for Practice Guidelines. J Am Coll Cardiol 2003;42:1687–713.

42. Montgomery JV, Harris KM. Relation of electrocardiographic patterns to phenotypic expression and clinical outcome in hypertrophic cardiomyopathy. Am J Cardiol 2005;96:270–5.

43. Ritter S, Tani LY, Etheridge SP, et al. What is the yield of screening echocardiography in pediatric syncope? Pediatrics 2000;105:E58.

44. Keren A, Syrris P, McKenna WJ. Hypertrophic cardiomyopathy: the genetic determinants of clinical disease expression. Nat Clin Pract Cardiovasc Med 2008;5(3): 158–68.

45. Colivicchi F, Ammirati F, Santini M. Epidemiology and prognostic implications of syncope in young competing athletes. Eur Heart J 2004;25:1749–53.
46. Tan HL, Hofman N, van Langen IM, et al. Sudden unexplained death: heritability and diagnostic yield of cardiological and genetic examination in surviving relatives. Circulation 2005;112(2):207–13.
47. Tester DJ, Spoon DB, Valdivia HH, et al. Targeted mutational analysis of the RyR2-encoded cardiac ryanodine receptor in sudden unexplained death: a molecular autopsy of 49 medical examiner/coroner's cases. Mayo Clin Proc 2004;79:1380–4.
48. Tester DJ, Ackerman MJ. The role of molecular autopsy in unexplained sudden cardiac death. Curr Opin Cardiol 2006;21:166–72.
49. Leslie L, Cohen J, Newburger J, et al. The costs and benefits of targeted screening for causes of sudden cardiac death in children and adolescents. Circulation 2012;125(21):2621–9.

Concussion and Trauma in Young Athletes: Prevention, Treatment, and Return-to-Play

Rance McClain, DO

KEYWORDS

- Athlete • Concussion • Mild traumatic brain injury • Second impact syndrome
- Computerized neurocognitive assessment

KEY POINTS

- Relative risk of suffering concussion/mild traumatic brain injury in youth sports participation.
- Proper initial assessment of youth athletes suspected of suffering a concussion.
- The common symptoms during the postconcussion period.
- The proper method of determining an athlete's return-to-play status.
- Second impact syndrome and how can people minimize the risk of an athlete suffering a second impact injury.

Millions of school-aged children participate in sports activities annually. Athletes and parents understand that injuries can, and do, occur during sports participation. However, neither group often considers the risk of serious injury when participating in athletic competitions and practices. In 2012, over 1.35 million children under the age of 19 were taken to the emergency room for injuries that occurred during participation in athletic events.[1] In the last few years there has been a growing awareness and interest in 1 sports injury in particular. At the forefront of public awareness is the issue of concussion, which is considered a subset of traumatic brain injury (TBI). The definition, in its most recent form, was updated at the 4th International Conference on Concussion in Sport held in Zurich, Switzerland in 2012 (**Box 1**).[2]

Neither I, nor my spouse, received anything of benefit from the production of this material from any commercial or business entity.
Kansas City University of Medicine and Biosciences, College of Osteopathic Medicine, 1750 Independence Avenue, Kansas City, MO 64106, USA
E-mail address: rmcclain@kcumb.edu

Prim Care Clin Office Pract 42 (2015) 77–83
http://dx.doi.org/10.1016/j.pop.2014.09.005   primarycare.theclinics.com

> **Box 1**
> **Consensus statement on concussion in sports**
>
> Concussion is a brain injury and is defined as a complex pathophysiological process affecting the brain, induced by biomechanical forces. Several common features that incorporate clinical, pathologic, and biomechanical injury constructs that may be utilized in defining the nature of a concussive head injury.
>
> 1. Concussion may be caused either by a direct blow to the head, face, neck, or elsewhere on the body with an "impulsive' force transmitted to the head.
>
> 2. Concussion typically results in the rapid onset of short-lived impairment of neurologic function that resolves spontaneously. However, in some cases, symptoms and signs may evolve over a number of minutes to hours.
>
> 3. Concussion may result in neuropathological changes, but the acute clinical symptoms largely reflect a functional disturbance rather than a structural injury and, as such, no abnormality is seen on standard structural neuroimaging studies.
>
> 4. Concussion results in a graded set of clinical symptoms that may or may not involve loss of consciousness. Resolution of the clinical and cognitive symptoms typically follows a sequential course. However, it is important to note that in some cases symptoms may be prolonged.
>
> *From* McCrory P, Meeuwisse WH, Aubry M, et al. Consensus statement on concussion in sport: the 4th International Conference on Concussion in Sport, Zurich, November 2012. J Athl Train 2013;48(4):555; with permission.

Concussions occur on a daily basis in youth athletics. From 2001 to 2009, annual emergency department visits for TBI increased in number from 153,375 to 248,418, with the highest rates among males ages 10 to 19 years.[3] Within this age group, nearly half (47%) of the concussions occurred in the 12- to 15-year-old age group subset.[1] This is occurring in spite of continued advances in athletic equipment and new measures to ensure increased safety of youth sports participants.

Awareness of head injuries and concussions is increasing in the United States, most likely due to a combination of coverage of this topic in mass media and aggressive awareness campaigns by organizations such as the Centers for Disease Control and Prevention (CDC), the National Football League (NFL) and USA Football. Programs developed and supported by these organizations, such as "Heads Up Football,"[4] are making a concerted effort to make the public aware of methods to reduce the risk of youth participants sustaining concussions during participation.

Efforts within each state have also occurred because of enactment of the Lystedt Laws.[5] These bills have been enacted as a follow-up to the state of Washington putting a bill in place in 2009 to protect young athletes from life-threatening or potentially lifelong consequences of returning to play too soon after sustaining a head injury. As of February 2014, all 50 states have put a similar law in place.[5] The original Lystedt Law was done in honor of Zackery Lystedt, a 13-year-old middle school football player who suffered permanent brain injury when he returned to play after suffering a concussion.[5]

The initial step in caring for concussed athletes is to develop an emergency action plan that includes a concussion protocol, which consists of recognition of injury, assessment, disposition, follow-up, return to play (RTP), and education.[6] Education efforts should include all persons around an athlete's participation such as the athletes themselves, their coaches, their parents, and the team trainers or physicians if available for the school or league.

Recognition of concussion can be complicated by the fact that many symptoms are not specific to concussion. The most common symptom, a headache, has many common causes. To establish a diagnosis of concussion, the headache should be correlated to a history of trauma to the head or body sufficient enough to transmit the force to the head. Signs and symptoms of a concussion include those in **Table 1**.[7]

Players often withhold this information. In 1 study by McCrea and colleagues, only 47.3% of high school football players with a concussion reported their injury. The reasoning behind their failure to report varied and included common reasoning of not thinking their symptoms were severe enough (66.4%), not wanting to be removed from play (41%), not realizing their symptoms were consistent with a concussion (36.1%) and not wanting to let their teammates down (22.1%).[8]

In addition to the recognition of signs and symptoms of concussion, other components to identifying concussed athletes include neurologic examination, balance assessment, and cognitive assessment. There are many standardized scales and checklists to achieve these assessments, with one of the most widely used being the Sports Concussion Assessment Tool—3rd Edition (SCAT3).[9] The developers also have a pediatric version for patients younger than 12 years of age in addition to the SCAT, named the Child SCAT3.[9]

In the last 20 years, there has been implementation and increasing usage of neuropsychological testing to assist in addressing the issue of identification and management of sports-related concussion.[10] These tests differ from sideline evaluation, in that they are designed to be given in the preseason period and are repeated when the athlete is asymptomatic after a concussive injury. It has been shown that symptoms of concussion often resolve before cognitive deficits, when measured with neuropsychological testing.[11] Neuropsychological tests represent another method to track patients after a concussive injury, but cannot be relied upon as a sole method of follow-up care for the concussed athlete.[12]

Table 1
Signs and symptoms of a concussion

Symptoms	Signs
• Headache	• Appears dazed
• Pressure in head	• Vacant facial expression
• Nausea or vomiting	• Confused about assignment
• Neck pain	• Forgets plays
• Balance problems or dizziness	• Is unsure of game, score, or opponent
• Blurred, double, or fuzzy vision	• Moves clumsily or displays incoordination
• Sensitivity to light or noise	• Answers questions slowly
• Feeling sluggish or slowed down	• Slurred speech
• Feeling foggy or groggy	• Shows behavior or personality changes
• Drowsiness	• Cannot recall events prior to hit
• Change in sleep pattern	• Cannot recall events after hit
• Amnesia	• Seizures or convulsions
• "Patient does not feel right"	• Any change in typical behavior or personality
• Fatigue or low energy	• Loses consciousness
• Sadness	
• Nervousness or anxiety	
• Irritability	
• More emotional	
• Confusion	
• Concentration or memory problems (forgetting game plays)	
• Repeating the same question/comment	

From Chrisman SP, Quitiquit C, Rivara FP. Qualitative study of barriers to concussive symptom reporting in high school athletics. J Adolesc Health 2013;52(3):330–5; with permission.

When an athlete is suspected as having a concussion, due to the presence of typical signs and symptoms after suffering trauma consistent with the development of a concussion, a decision must be made as to that athlete's disposition. The current recommendation is that no athlete who is suspected as to have suffered a concussive injury be allowed to return to play that day.[2] This is a more aggressive stance than previously utilized and is a direct response attempting to protect athletes, in particular young athletes, from second impact syndrome (SIS). Nearly all cases of second impact syndrome occurred in high school athletes and adolescents.[13]

SIS is a rare, often fatal, TBI that occurs when a repeat injury is sustained before symptoms of a previous head injury have resolved.[14] The pathophysiology of SIS is poorly understood, but has been attributed to loss of autoregulation and resultant massive swelling of the brain, potentially resulting in herniation. Authors have hypothesized that this disruption of autoregulation occurs as a result of reinjury to neuronal cells during a vulnerable period of ongoing internal derangement from a previous injury.[15] A second aspect to the original hypothesis was the thought that there were likely space-occupying injuries that were present within the head as part of the original injury. However, Weinstein and colleagues[16] demonstrated, in a single case study, that no space-occupying injuries occurred at a detectable level on a computed tomography (CT) scan of a 17-year-old high school football player who suffered an SIS injury.

Most athletes in the acute period following a concussion can be observed and managed with conservative care. However, there are situations when an athlete needs to be sent for emergency evaluation. Cases involving deteriorating mental status or worsening symptoms are of particular concern. Specific symptoms that raise concern include worsening headache, nausea or vomiting, or increasing lethargy. Worsening symptoms such as these necessitate transport to a facility that can handle neurosurgical emergencies.[17] Historically, these types of decisions, as well as return to play decisions, were loosely based on the grading of concussion severity. Recently, organizations are doing away with grading systems, and are attempting to individualize the approach to each athlete.[18]

Once an athlete is felt to have recovered from his or her concussive injury and be fit for return to play consideration, it is best to use a graduated stepwise approach. **Table 2** represents the most recent guidelines as defined in the consensus statement on concussion in sport. Each phase should take approximately 24 hours to progress through, and the athlete must remain asymptomatic during the activities at that phase. If an athlete has symptoms while attempting activities within a phase, he or she is instructed to rest for 24 hours, then drop down to the previous phase and resume activity at that level. If he or she is again symptomatic at that level, activity can be increased up a level and continued on as long as symptom free.[2]

Most concussions are mild and self-limited, and the symptoms go away within approximately 1 week. However, occasionally symptoms of a concussion can persist for weeks or months. On rare occasions, symptoms can persist and become permanent following a concussion. One study of sports-related concussion in high school athletes showed that 50% of the athletes recovered and returned to play in 1 week, and by 3 weeks after concussion, 83% had returned to play. Seventeen percent of athletes had symptoms that persisted longer than 3 weeks.[19] Of particular concern, it has been shown in research studies that younger athletes had a longer mean time to recovery when compared with older athletes.[20]

Studies have been conducted to attempt to identify signs or symptoms that would predict a prolonged recovery time. Athletes who present with 4 or more symptoms were 2 times more likely to have symptoms that lasted more than 7 days. They also

Table 2
Graduated return to play protocol

Rehabilitation Stage	Functional Exercise at Each Stage of Rehabilitation	Objective of Each Stage
1. No activity	Symptom limited physical and cognitive rest	Recovery
2. Light aerobic exercise	Walking, swimming, or stationary cycling keeping intensity <70% maximum permitted heart rate No resistance training	Increase heart rate
3. Sport-specific exercise	Skating drills in ice hockey, running drills in soccer No head impact activities	Add movement
4. Noncontact training drills	Progression to more complex training drills, (eg, passing drills in football and ice hockey) May start progressive resistance training	Exercise, coordination, and cognitive load
5. Full-contact practice	Following medical clearance participate in normal training activities	Restore confidence and assess functional skills by coaching staff
6. Return to play	Normal game play	

From McCrory P, Meeuwisse WH, Aubry M, et al. Consensus statement on concussion in sport: the 4th International Conference on Concussion in Sport, Zurich, November 2012. J Athl Train 2013;48(4):554–75; with permission.

concluded that athletes who reported feeling drowsy or had nausea or confusion with concentration difficulties at the time of injury were more likely to have concussion symptoms that lasted more than 7 days.[21] A study by McCrea and colleagues showed a prolonged recovery (>7 days) was associated with unconsciousness, post-traumatic amnesia, and more severe acute symptoms.[22] In another study, a higher total score on a Post-Concussion Symptom Scale (PCSS) was associated with symptoms persisting more than 28 days. However, that study failed to show a statistically significant relationship between loss of consciousness or amnesia and prolonged symptoms of more than 28 days.[23]

Other aspects of postconcussion syndrome have been identified, even after just 1 concussive injury. Kontos followed concussed high school and collegiate athletes for 2 weeks after concussion. He identified elevated levels of depression in athletes at 2 days, 7 days and 14 days after concussion in all athletes. The increase in depression levels persisted at both the 7- and 14-day evaluations, even after controlling for nondepressive symptoms.[24] Another study, done on adolescents, showed a decrease in peak anterior velocity of the center of mass (COM) and had more significant medial/lateral COM displacement when walking while performing a concurrent cognitive task.[25] This balance problem could be of particular concern in adolescent athletes, as they are required to process their surroundings cognitively while the event is occurring. A decreased anterior velocity and increased medial/lateral COM displacement could increase an athlete's chances of becoming injured.

One of the most concerning aspects of concussion, and one that has garnered an increased amount of media attention in the last several decades is the risk of chronic neurodegenerative changes with recurrent head trauma. The list of conditions includes chronic traumatic encephalopathy (CTE), mild cognitive impairment, and dementia pugilistica. The pathologic findings of CTE include progressive tauopathy and axonal loss of varying degrees of severity and range from focal to diffuse changes.[26] The clinical symptoms of CTE begin after a long period of latency ranging from several years to several decades. The initial symptoms are typically insidious, consisting of irritability, impulsivity, aggression, depression, short-term memory loss and heightened suicidality. The symptoms progress slowly over decades to include cognitive deficits and dementia.[27]

SUMMARY

The risk to any individual pediatric athlete suffering a concussion is relatively low. It is vitally important for athletes, as well as anyone in contact with athletes, to be able to recognize the signs and symptoms of concussion. Only when there are plans for the identification and treatment of concussions can the athletes be fully protected and properly cared for. These plans must include the athlete, parents, coach(es), teachers, and anyone else who has a role in the athlete's daily activities following a concussive episode. It is this vigilance to a proper follow-up and treatment protocol that can potentially reduce the rates of prolonged postconcussion symptoms and decrease the likelihood of any morbidity and mortality associated with concussions in pediatric athletes.

REFERENCES

1. Ferguson RW. Safe kids worldwide analysis of CPSC NEISS data. Bethesda (MD): National Electronic Injury Surveillance System; 2013.
2. McCrory P, Meeuwisse WH, Aubry M, et al. Consensus statement on concussion in sport: the 4th International Conference on Concussion in Sport, Zurich, November 2012. J Athl Train 2013;48(4):554–75.
3. Centers for Disease Control and Prevention. Nonfatal traumatic brain injuries related to sports and recreation activities among persons aged ≤19 years-United States, 2001–2009. MMWR Morb Mortal Wkly Rep 2011;60:1337–42.
4. Available at: http://usafootball.com/headsup. Accessed March 13, 2014.
5. Available at: http://www.nflevolution.com/article/The-Zackery-Lystedt-Law?ref=270. Accessed March 13, 2014.
6. Herring SA, Cantu RC, Guskiewicz KM, et al, American College of Sports Medicine. Concussion (mild traumatic brain injury) and the team physician: a consensus statement—2011 update. Med Sci Sports Exerc 2011;43(12):2412–22.
7. Chrisman SP, Quitiquit C, Rivara FP. Qualitative study of barriers to concussive symptom reporting in high school athletics. J Adolesc Health 2013;52(3):330–5.
8. McCrea M, Hammeke T, Olsen G, et al. Unreported concussion in high school football players: implications for prevention. Clin J Sport Med 2004;14(1):13–7.
9. Available at: http://download.lww.com/wolterskluwer_vitalstream_com/PermaLink/JSM/A/JSM_23_2_2013_02_14_MCCRORYY_200872_SDC2.pdf. Accessed March 14, 2014.
10. Echemendia RJ. Sports neuropsychology: assessment and management of traumatic brain injury. New York: Guilford Press; 2006.
11. Echemendia R, Putukian M, Mackin RS, et al. Neuropsychological test performance prior to and following sports-related mild traumatic brain injury. Clin J Sport Med 2001;11:23–31.

12. Randolph C, McCrea M, Barr WB. Is neuropsychological testing useful in the medical management of sport-related concussion? J Athl Train 2005;40(3): 136–51.
13. Pellman EJ, Viano DC. Concussion in professional football: summary of the research conducted by the National Football League's Committee on Mild Traumatic Brain Injury. Neurosurg Focus 2006;21(4):E12.
14. Cantu RC. Second Impact Syndrome. Clin Sports Med 1998;17:37–44.
15. McCrory P. Does second impact syndrome exist? Clin J Sport Med 2001;11: 144–9.
16. Weinstein E, Turner M, Kuzma BB, et al. Second impact syndrome in football: new imaging and insights into a rare and devastating condition. J Neurosurg Pediatr 2013;11(3):331–4.
17. Putukian M. The acute symptoms of sport-related concussion: diagnosis and on-field management. Clin Sports Med 2011;30:49–61.
18. Available at: https://www.aan.com/uploadedFiles/Website_Library_Assets/Docu ments/3Practice_Management/5Patient_Resources/1For_Your_Patient/6_Sports_ Concussion_Toolkit/guidelines.pdf. Accessed March 14, 2014.
19. Collins MW, Lovell MR, Iverson GL, et al. Examining concussion rates and return to play in high school football players wearing newer helmet technology: at three-year prospective study. Neurosurgery 2006;58(2):275–86.
20. Field M, Collins MW, Lovell MR, et al. Does age play a role in recovery from sports-related concussion? A comparison of high school and collegiate athletes. J Pediatr 2003;142:546–53.
21. Chrisman SP, Rivara FP, Schiff MA, et al. Risk factors for concussive symptoms 1 week or longer in high school athletes. Brain Inj 2013;27(1):1–9.
22. McCrea M, Guskiewicz K, Randoph C, et al. Incidence, clinical course and predictors of prolonged recovery time following sport-related concussion in high school and college athletes. J Int Neuropsychol 2013;19(1):22–33.
23. Meehan WE 3rd, Mannix RC, Stracciolini A, et al. Symptom severity predicts prolonged recovery after sport-related concussion, but age and amnesia do not. J Pediatr 2013;163(3):721–55.
24. Kontos AP, Covassin T, Elbin RJ, et al. Depression and neurocognitive performance after concussion among male and female high school and collegiate athletes. Arch Phys Med Rehabil 2012;93(10):1751–6.
25. Howell DR, Osternig LR, Chou LS. Dual-task effect on gait balance control in adolscents with concussion. Arch Phys Med Rehabil 2013;94(8):1513–20.
26. Tartaglia MC, Hazrati LN, Davis KD, et al. Chronic traumatic encephalopathy and other neurodegenerative proteinopathies. Front Hum Neurosci 2014;8:30.
27. Stein TD, Alvarex VE, McKee AC. Chronic traumatic encephalopathy: a spectrum of neuropathological changes following repetitive brain trauma in athletes and military personnel. Alzheimers Res Ther 2014;6(1):4.

Care of Children with Autism Spectrum Disorder

Kathryn Ellerbeck, MD*, Catherine Smith, PhD, Andrea Courtemanche, PhD

KEYWORDS

- Autism spectrum disorder • Physician's role • Medical home
- Co-occurring conditions

KEY POINTS

- Physicians play an important role in the identification of children with possible autism spectrum disorder (ASD).
- Children with ASD often have co-occurring medical, mental health, and educational needs.
- Physicians need to refer children and families for appropriate diagnosis and treatment.
- Physicians should provide a medical home for the child with ASD.

INTRODUCTION

Autism Is Common and Complex

Recent data from the Centers for Disease Control and Prevention (CDC) and the Autism and Developmental Disabilities Monitoring (ADDM) network estimate that by age 8 years, 1 in every 68 children has a diagnosis of autism spectrum disorder (ASD). The average age of diagnosis for children has remained stable at 4.5 years of age.[1] Children having adequate language and cognitive skills are often not diagnosed until they enter school. As a result, many primary care physicians (PCPs) will be faced with the question "Doctor, does my child have autism?"

Diagnostic Criteria for Autism Spectrum Disorder

In addition to being common, ASD is also complex. In May 2013, new diagnostic criteria for ASD were published in the *Diagnostic and Statistical Manual of Mental Disorders*, 5th edition (DSM-5).[2] The DSM-5 is a manual that presents a classification of mental disorders and diagnostic criteria used to identify and diagnose mental disorders. Perhaps the most notable change in the DSM-5 ASD criteria is the elimination of ASD subtypes (Asperger Syndrome, Autistic Disorder, Pervasive Developmental

The authors have no conflicts of interest to disclose.
Center for Child Health and Development, University of Kansas Medical Center, 3901 Rainbow Blvd. MS 4003, Kansas City, KS 66160, USA
* Corresponding author.
E-mail address: kellerbeck@kumc.edu

Disorder, Not Otherwise Specified,(PDD_NOS), Childhood Disintegrative Disorder). The new DSM-5 criteria allow for a single categorical diagnosis of ASD. The diagnostic criteria are now combined into 2 core symptom areas: deficits in social relatedness and social communication, and repetitive and restricted patterns of behavior. However, the behaviors and symptoms that were previously used to diagnose ASD are largely the same. Autism is still autism. The DSM-5 recommends that the diagnostician identify "specifiers" about the individual with ASD, so that providers will have a better understanding of areas of strength and needs. The DSM-5 diagnostic criteria for ASD can be found in the DSM-5[2] or at http://www.cdc.gov/ncbddd/autism/hcp-dsm.html.

A diagnosis of ASD is given when individuals meet *all 3 criteria* in the area of deficits in social communication/social interaction, and *at least 2 criteria* in the area of repetitive and restricted behaviors/interests. Symptoms must be present in early childhood, cause significant impairment in functioning, and are not better accounted for by intellectual disability or global developmental delay. Recent changes to ASD criteria in the DSM-5 should not affect individuals previously diagnosed with an ASD using the *Diagnostic and Statistical Manual of Mental Disorders*, 4th edition, Text Revision, (DSM-IV-TR).[3] According to the DSM-5, if an individual was diagnosed using the DSM-IV-TR, he or she is considered to meet ASD criteria using DSM-5; therefore, diagnoses given using DSM-IV are not being removed based on the new criteria (**Box 1**).[2]

Roles for the Primary Care Physician

The primary care physician (PCP) plays a vital role for children with ASD. This article focuses on the roles of PCPs in the Medical Home, which include:

1. Performing developmental surveillance, screening, and referral
2. Assisting in the diagnostic process
3. Identifying and managing co-occurring conditions
4. Supporting children and families across systems

MEDICAL HOMES FOR CHILDREN WITH AUTISM SPECTRUM DISORDER

Pediatricians and PCPs are likely to be familiar with the definition and principles of the family-centered (or patient-centered) medical home.[4–6] The pediatric medical home is "a model of delivering primary medical care that is accessible, continuous, comprehensive, family-centered, coordinated, compassionate, and culturally effective."[5]

Box 1
Major changes to the DSM-5, Autism Diagnostic Criteria

Major Changes to the DSM-5 Include:

Category name changed from Pervasive Developmental Disorders to Autism Spectrum Disorders

- Elimination of specific ASD subtypes (Asperger Syndrome, PDD-NOS, Autistic Disorder, Childhood Disintegration Disorder) and a move to one diagnosis, Autism Spectrum Disorder

- Reduction/combination of core symptoms categories from 3 to 2 (socialization and communication are now one combined category, repetitive and restricted behaviors/interests). Inclusion of sensory differences in criteria

- Recommendation to identify "specifiers" to better understand the individual needs of each child with ASD (cognitive and language ability, level of supports needed, co-occurring medical and mental health conditions)

- Inclusion of co-occurring mental health disorders (eg, attention-deficit/hyperactivity disorder)

However, PCPs may be less familiar with building a medical home for children with ASD. Children with ASD are less likely to be served in a medical home.[7] A medical home for children with ASD requires substantial collaboration and coordination across systems, and may be more complicated than medical homes for children with other chronic conditions.[8] A physician survey found that physicians feel less competent in caring for children with ASD (and other neurodevelopmental conditions) than with children with other chronic medical conditions.[9] In a series of focus groups, Carbone and colleagues[10] explored the perspectives of parents and pediatricians with regard to caring for children with ASD within the medical home. Carbone found parents to be unfamiliar with the concept of medical home. After defining it, he found that parents of children with ASD did not expect to receive help with comprehensive and coordinated care from their physicians, and believed that their physicians were unlikely to be able to provide the services described. Physicians understood what the families of children with ASD faced, but considered themselves ill-prepared to meet the array of needs (**Box 2**).

PERFORMING DEVELOPMENTAL SURVEILLANCE, SCREENING, AND REFERRAL

Although this article focuses on ASD in the school-age child, many families note symptoms years earlier. The diagnostic journey for families of children with possible ASD is often difficult, time-consuming, and expensive.[11,12] Families are often frustrated by their physicians' lack of attention to red-flag symptoms for ASD, and report that referral for diagnosis and treatment is often delayed months or years following initial reported concerns.[5,7,13-15] Although ASD symptoms can be recognized at or before the age of 2 years in most children, the average age at which a child receives an ASD diagnosis is 4.5 years (**Box 3**).[1]

With the growing evidence that early intervention improves developmental outcomes for even very young children,[16] much of the focus by the American Academy of Pediatrics (AAP) has been on autism surveillance and screening in toddlers. A significant percentage of children, however, either are not screened as toddlers or do not have symptoms that can be clearly recognized until school-age, when universal screening is no longer recommended (**Box 4**).

Identification of the child with developmental delays and/or autism symptoms is recognized to be part of the physician's responsibility in providing well child care.[17] Physicians often hold the keys to access evidence-based interventions that yield the best outcomes for the futures of children with ASD.[18] In 2007, the AAP published 2 clinical reports on ASD. The first, *Identification and Evaluation of Children with Autism Spectrum Disorder* (http://pediatrics.aappublications.org/content/120/5/1183.full) provides background information and an algorithm to help PCPs develop

---

Box 2
AAP guidelines for surveillance and screening

"Surveillance entails asking parents at every well-child visit about developmental or behavioral concerns, observing for early signs of autism, and documenting a family history of ASDs."

"Screening involves administering an autism-specific test to all children at their 18- and 24- [or 30-] month office visits, not just to children who demonstrate autistic behaviors."

From Carbone PS, Farley M, Davis T. Primary care for children with autism. Am Fam Physician 2010;8:453–60.

Box 3
Possible red flags for ASD

A child with ASD might:

- Not respond to their name by 12 months of age
- Not point at objects to show interest (point at an airplane flying over) by 14 months
- Not play "pretend" games (pretend to "feed" a doll) by 18 months
- Avoid eye contact and want to be alone
- Have trouble understanding other people's feelings or talking about their own feelings
- Have delayed speech and language skills
- Repeat words or phrases over and over (echolalia)
- Give unrelated answers to questions
- Get upset by minor changes
- Have obsessive interests
- Flap their hands, rock their body, or spin in circles
- Have unusual reactions to the way things sound, smell, taste, look, or feel

From Centers for Disease Control and Prevention. Autism spectrum disorder. Signs and symptoms. Available at: http://www.cdc.gov/ncbddd/autism/signs.html. Accessed September 19, 2014.

Box 4
ASD symptoms in the school-age child

Doctor, Does My Child Have Autism?

Symptoms in the School-Age Child

My child…

- Has no friends
- Likes to play alone
- Has poor eye contact
- Repeats lines from TV
- Cannot carry on a conversation
- Has intense interests that occupy all of his/her time
- Lines up his/her toys
- Does strange things with his/her hands
- Has to have things a certain way
- Only talks about his/her interests
- Has difficulty with changes in routines
- Gets teased
- Has problems with transitioning from activity to activity
- Is a picky eater and will only eat certain types and textures of foods
- Has extreme tantrums
- Does not understand social cues

a strategy for early identification of children with ASD.[19] Pediatricians are to incorporate developmental surveillance at every well child visit, and conduct routine screening of all infants for ASD at the 18-month and 24- or 30-month visits, as well as at any visit that a parent raises concern. Children who fail autism screens are to be referred both to the early intervention system and to developmental specialists for definitive diagnosis of ASD. At present, the AAP does not recommend universal screening for school-age children. However, there are some evidence-based screening tools that can help determine whether further evaluation is needed. For a review of characteristics of some of the school-age screening tools, see Norris and Lecavalier[20] (**Table 1**).

The Primary Care Physician's Role in the Diagnosis of Autism Spectrum Disorder

Beyond screening, who can diagnose ASDs? There is substantial variability of symptoms, which makes diagnostic decision-making challenging. Definitive diagnosis of ASD may be beyond the scope of primary care practice. The AAP recommends that children identified as being at risk for a diagnosis of ASD be referred for a comprehensive developmental and diagnostic assessment. ASD diagnosis is often given by pediatric subspecialists such as developmental-behavioral pediatricians, neurologists, child psychiatrists, or licensed psychologists. Expertise in the area of ASD has been found to be more important to accurate diagnosis than particular credentials.[19,21,22] The insurance systems in many states, however, require that a medical diagnosis of ASD be given only by a physician or psychologist.[18]

Medical Diagnosis of Autism Spectrum Disorder

A medical diagnosis of ASD is something of a misnomer. Autism is not "a disease," but rather a behaviorally defined disorder resulting from atypical development of the immature brain.[23] Use of the term medical diagnosis conflates categorical DSM-5 diagnosis and etiologic diagnosis. Both are important, but each requires PCPs to collaborate with different groups of specialists.

Although children with ASD by definition have deficits in social communication, social interaction and restricted, repetitive patterns of behavior, there is a wide spectrum of symptom presentation and severity. Unfortunately, there is no biological marker that predicts the DSM-5 diagnosis of ASD. Best practices in ASD diagnostic evaluation require the assessment of multiple areas of functioning. A comprehensive evaluation must include a parent interview and an observation of the child's current functioning by a clinician experienced with ASD.[24]

Table 1 ASD screening tools for the school-age child		
Screening Tool	**Age Range (y)**	**How to Access?**
Social Communication Questionnaire (SCQ)	4 to adult	www.wpspublish.com
Social Responsiveness Scale (SRS)	4–18	www.wpspublish.com
Autism Spectrum Screening Questionnaire (ASSQ)	7–16	http://scatn.med.sc.edu/screening/ehlers-assq-1999[1].pdf
Childhood Autism Spectrum Test (CAST)	4–11	http://www.autismresearchcentre.com/arc_tests

As per AAP recommendations, physicians who are providing care for a child with symptoms of autism are to refer to developmental specialists or interdisciplinary autism diagnostic teams, which are often located within urban, university-based settings. Follow through with these referrals may be problematic given that subspecialty services are limited in number and may not be accessible to rural and underserved populations. Furthermore, wait times for diagnostic evaluations at specialized diagnostic centers are long and may exceed 9 to 12 months, thus delaying children's diagnosis of ASD.[18] However, this should neither delay the assessment of the child in the educational system nor the treatment of co-occurring conditions in the medical home. Both families and physicians need to be aware that children may be eligible for an educational identification of Autism and for special education services through the public school district without having a clinical DSM-5 diagnosis of ASD. The school district can complete an educational evaluation to determine the child's need for special education services and support through the development of an Individualized Education Plan (IEP). Families may be told that a "private" or "medical" diagnosis of ASD is required for the child to be eligible for educational support. However, this is not true, and violates the requirements of the Individuals with Disabilities Education Act (IDEA).[17]

The PCP is not well positioned to determine whether the child meets DSM-5 criteria for ASD. However, the PCP has a significant role in the child's medical management. Every child with cognitive impairment and/or suspected ASD should see a physician with the aim of finding the underlying cause of the developmental problems. Diagnosing the underlying cause for ASD may require the PCP to coordinate genetic testing and referral to a genetic subspecialist.

IDENTIFYING AND MANAGING CO-OCCURRING CONDITIONS

Children with ASD have the same basic health needs as typically developing children, but are significantly more likely than other children to have a variety of medical and psychiatric symptoms and diagnoses, more frequent physician visits, and to be prescribed psychotropic medication.[25–28] The second Clinical Report published by the AAP in 2007 was *Management of Children with Autism Spectrum Disorder* (http://pediatrics.aappublications.org/content/120/5/1162.full). This report provides guidance to PCPs on management of the child with ASD in the medical home.

Physicians in the medical home should provide medical care and, when necessary, refer to subspecialty medical care. PCPs are also in the position to direct families to appropriate behavioral specialists for disruptive or maladaptive behavior (**Box 5**).[8,27]

Box 5
Physician's roles: identifying and managing co-occurring conditions

- Review commonly presenting medical issues that co-occur in ASD, including seizure, gastrointestinal symptoms and dietary restrictions, and sleep disorders. Consult with necessary medical subspecialists.

- Review commonly presenting behavioral/psychiatric issues that co-occur in ASD, including attention-deficit/hyperactivity disorder, anxiety, obsessive-compulsive disorder, mood disorder, and disruptive behavior. Consult with necessary behavioral subspecialists.

- Collaborate with both medical and behavioral specialists with regard to medication management of co-occurring symptoms.

Physician Roles in Managing Medical Co-Occurring Conditions

Seizures, gastrointestinal problems, and sleep disturbance are commonly reported by parents of children with ASD, and can cause both children and families considerable distress.[19,29]

- Seizures occur in approximately 25% to 30% of individuals with ASD. Children who have developmental delay or intellectual disability associated with their ASD are at particularly high risk for seizures. Just as for typically developing children who have seizures, PCPs may need to consult child neurologists regarding medication management.[19,29]
- There has been debate about the frequency and nature of gastrointestinal disorders in children with ASD.[29] Children with ASD with gastrointestinal symptoms deserve the same thorough diagnostic evaluation as a child who does not have ASD.[30] Problem behaviors can occur because of underlying gastrointestinal symptoms. Children with ASD can have very restricted eating, and may have more constipation than children with a more normal diet. Treatment of constipation can improve toilet training and decrease disruptive behaviors.[10,25,29–31]
- Sleep disorders are more common in children with ASD than in typically developing children.[8,10,32] Melatonin is often effective for sleep-onset disorders in children with ASD[33] and seems to be safe. PCPs should become comfortable with prescribing melatonin. Children who have severe sleep problems and fail to respond to behavioral interventions or melatonin may benefit from being evaluated in a sleep disorders clinic.

Physician Roles in Managing Behavioral Co-Occurring Conditions

Children with ASD often have co-occurring disruptive behavior and may meet criteria for co-occurring psychiatric diagnoses.[27,34,35] Tantrums and aggression are particularly difficult for families of children with ASD.[36] Children with ASD who have behavioral deterioration need to have a physical examination with consideration that pain or discomfort may be the cause. Physicians should work with behavioral specialists to identify the functions of disruptive behavior. Functional analysis of behavior can inform both appropriate behavioral intervention and medication management. Unfortunately, PCPs often have difficulty in finding appropriately trained mental health providers who can help determine the causes and treatments for disruptive behaviors and who will communicate regularly with the medical home.[36] Understanding which factors exacerbate or maintain the behavior is critically important to designing behavioral interventions, and may be important in determining appropriate use of psychotropic medications.[8] A handout from the AAP's 2012 Autism Toolkit on Behavioral Principles is available at http://www.medicalhomeinfo.org/downloads/pdfs/Behavioral%20Principles.F0620.pdf.

The PCP can expect to receive specific details about the child that support the diagnosis from the diagnostician.[24] The report should also include treatment recommendations that are specific to the child's autism symptoms and co-occurring conditions. The PCP will need to have some familiarity with commonly recommended evidence-based treatments.

One of the most requested evidenced-based treatments for ASD is applied behavior analysis (ABA).[37,38] ABA is based on the science of learning and behavior, and is one of the only scientifically based treatments for children with ASD.[39] ABA uses the "laws" of behavior to promote skill acquisition (eg, language, adaptive skills, and academic skills) and decrease unwanted behaviors (eg, aggression, self-injury, and repetitive behaviors). ABA interventions are structured and systematic. These interventions involve data collection on target skills and behaviors with the use of positive strategies for behavior change. ABA-based interventions may include discrete trial teaching, verbal behavior approaches, and pivotal response training. ABA providers can be found at http://bacb.com/. In addition, Autism Speaks has developed a parent toolkit describing ABA services. The toolkit can be downloaded at http://www.autismspeaks.org/family-services/tool-kits/.

Physician Roles in Managing Psychotropic Medications

There is still little evidence that medication effectively treats the social and communication impairments of ASD.[40,41] Although risperidone (Risperdal) and aripiprazole (Abilify) are approved by the Food and Drug Administration for ASD and have been shown to decrease irritability and disruptive behavior, a substantial percentage of children on atypical neuroleptics experience excessive weight gain, limiting the use of these medications.[42,43] PCPs may or may not be comfortable with medicating the symptoms of attention-deficit/hyperactivity disorder (ADHD) and anxiety that frequently co-occur with ASD. Many physicians may consult psychiatrists or developmental-behavioral pediatricians who are more familiar with medications. Given the limited access families often have to developmental-behavioral pediatricians and psychiatrists, PCPs may need to collaborate with these subspecialists to prescribe and manage psychotropic medications (**Box 6**).[8,10]

BARRIERS TO THE PRIMARY CARE PHYSICIAN'S ROLE
Barriers to Adoption of Best Practices in the Diagnosis of Children with Autism Spectrum Disorder

As already noted, there is a lack of clarity with regard to what is meant by screening, educational identification, and clinical diagnosis of ASD among both the educational and the broader health care systems, creating a disconnect between the systems.[22] The disconnect between the health care, educational, and family systems frequently results in delayed diagnosis of ASD because symptoms are initially overlooked or misdiagnosed. Children in rural or underserved populations are often diagnosed later because of limited access to diagnostic services and the lack of knowledge and experience with ASD across these systems.[44]

Barriers to Adoption of Best Practices in Early Identification of Children with Autism Spectrum Disorder

Physicians face significant challenges in adopting best practices. It has only been over the last 15 to 20 years that ASD has been recognized to be a common, rather than an uncommon disorder.[45] Many physicians still receive little training about ASD. Families, physicians, and educators may have confusion over the roles that PCPs should play in

---

Box 6
CDC resources

The Centers for Disease Control and Prevention (CDC) has published a free resource to help PCPs with identification and management of children with ASD. *Autism Case Training: Specific Anticipatory Guidance* is available at: http://www.cdc.gov/ncbddd/actearly/autism/case-modules/anticipatory-guidance/page3b.html.

the diagnostic process. If the PCP is unable to make a clinical diagnosis of ASD based on DSM-5 criteria, it is appropriate to refer the child for a more comprehensive diagnosis. Unfortunately, autism diagnostic teams often have long wait lists, leading to lengthy delays between a failed screen and definitive diagnosis, thus increasing parent and physician level of frustration and anxiety.[18] Families of children who fail autism screening tools often wait months between screening and appointments for definitive diagnosis. During this time, these families will need ongoing support from the medical home.

Barriers to Adoption of Best Practices in Management of Co-Occurring Conditions

There are barriers to providing optimal care to children with ASD.

- Communication impairment often limits the child's ability to communicate discomfort, and difficult behaviors may make adequate physical examination difficult.
- The complexity of ASD warrants collaboration across systems (ie, medical, mental health, educational, family, and community), which can be complicated.
- Parents may also have beliefs about the cause of the child's autism that physicians do not share, which may adversely affect the family's relationship with the medical home. Parent refusal or delay of vaccines is common and particularly challenging for many physicians.[9,46,47] Many, if not most families of children with ASD also use complementary and alternative medicine (CAM). Physicians feel inadequately prepared to discuss CAM, and report the CAM use is a barrier to providing primary care.[9,48] Families and physicians may disagree about the use of CAM, and many popular treatments have not been well studied and have limited evidence for efficacy.[49] However, it is important to understand parental beliefs. The AAP recommends family-centered care, which includes open communication and sensitivity when managing differences around immunizations, treatments, and philosophy.[9] The CDC and AAP have developed resources to support physicians and educate families as they negotiate differences in beliefs.[50,51]

OPPORTUNITIES TO SUPPORT CHILDREN AND FAMILIES ACROSS SYSTEMS

This article highlights the vital role of the PCP in identifying, managing, and supporting school-age children with ASD within the medical home. Gaining familiarity with symptom presentation, course, and the most recent DSM-5 diagnostic criteria for ASD will help PCPs recognize this disorder in the school-age population they serve. Once the concern for ASD is raised, the PCP should then refer for diagnostic evaluation by an autism specialist and evaluation by the child's educational team.[24] These 2 referrals are the most important the PCP can make to ensure the child receives an accurate diagnosis and appropriate educational and behavioral services. The diagnostic process may be a long and stressful, and families will require support from their PCP. One way to reduce stress is to refer the child for intervention to treat specific symptoms while the child is waiting for the diagnostic evaluation. For example, the child may benefit from a referral to community behavioral and mental health agencies to address symptoms that commonly occur with ASD (eg, anxiety, depression, behavior problems, activity level). As mentioned earlier, the educational team should not wait on clinical diagnoses before beginning the evaluation process to determine if the child is eligible for special education services. Making these referrals will help support families while they wait for a definitive diagnosis of ASD.

The PCP should expect to receive a report from the autism diagnosticians that fully describes the individual with ASD in terms of symptom severity, cognition and language abilities, and co-occurring medical and behavioral conditions. This information should guide the PCP in providing optimum care for the school-age child with ASD in the medical home. In summary, PCPs plays an integral role in the identification, management, and care for their patients with ASD. The following case illustrates the key points of this article.

Case in Point

Caitlyn is an 8-year-old girl who is in the second grade and has experienced some difficulty with learning to read. She does not have an IEP through the public school system. Caitlyn's 2-year-old brother has severe developmental delays, and you had referred him for evaluation, including genetic testing. He was just diagnosed with Fragile X syndrome. Caitlyn's parents are overwhelmed with the needs of both children. Caitlyn is noncompliant, has frequent tantrums, and has difficulties with completing her homework. Although she has fewer disruptive behaviors at school, at the recent Parent-Teacher meeting her parents were told that Caitlyn has attention problems, is anxious with any change to daily routine, and is very rude to her classmates. Caitlyn seems to want friends, but she is rarely included in any play at recess. Caitlyn's parents tell you that she is never invited to activities outside of school. Caitlyn's parents need some help, and ask what they should do next.

You think that Caitlyn's problems may be related to her learning problems or possibly ADHD, but you are concerned about the school's report of social problems. You ask Caitlyn's parents to complete the Childhood Autism Screening Test (CAST). The score on the CAST suggests referral for a comprehensive autism evaluation. You refer Caitlyn to the nearest autism diagnostic center, which is 3 hours away.

Question 1
Given the concerns, does Caitlyn need to "fail" a screen to be referred?

Answer 1
No. Although the CAST may help you discuss your concerns with Caitlyn's parents who are just adjusting to their son's diagnosis and who have no knowledge of autism, the school's concerns about Caitlyn's social difficulties and problems with transition is sufficient reason for referral.

After you complete the referral, Caitlyn's parents complete the required paperwork, and are told that the wait list for the diagnostic center is approximately 6 months. As a result of her brother's Fragile X diagnosis, Caitlyn is also tested and also is found to have Fragile X syndrome. Caitlyn was suspended from school for 3 days because she attacked a teacher.

Question 2
Which of the following would be the most appropriate next step for Caitlyn and her family?

A. Tell the family that it is likely that Fragile X syndrome explains Caitlyn's behaviors, and refer the family to the local Fragile X support group. Cancel the autism diagnostic evaluation appointment.
B. Ask the school to do complete psychoeducational testing to look at Caitlyn's learning strengths and weaknesses, and to determine whether Caitlyn needs an IEP.
C. Wait for the recommendations from the autism diagnostic clinic appointment before doing any more referrals, because you know that Fragile X syndrome can be associated with ASD.

D. Refer the family to a behavioral therapist who has expertise in treating children with ADHD and oppositional behaviors.

E. B and D

Answer 2

E. Although the underlying etiology for Caitlyn's learning and behavioral problems is likely to be Fragile X syndrome, she needs an evaluation to determine whether she meets DSM-5 criteria for ASD, ADHD, anxiety, and/or possible learning disabilities. The school has a responsibility to determine whether Caitlyn needs educational supports. As there is a concern about ASD, it might be helpful to advocate for an autism educational specialist to be involved. Caitlyn also has very challenging behaviors at home and at school, and her family would benefit from working with a therapist who could help them manage her challenging behaviors. You could also help by assisting in an evaluation to see whether Caitlyn may have ADHD symptoms that could potentially respond to medication management.

Caitlyn is seen by the autism diagnostic team. As per best practice recommendations, the autism diagnostic team includes information from your office, from Caitlyn's school, and from her family. The team administers gold-standard autism diagnostic tools, which include a parent interview [Autism Diagnostic Interview-Revised (ADI-R)] and a play-based assessment (Autism Diagnostic Observation Schedule, Second Edition, ADOS-2). Their impressions are as follows:

1. Meets DSM-5 Criteria for ASD
   Severity of social communication: Level 1 (requires support)
   Severity of restricted, repetitive behaviors: Level 2 (requires substantial support)
2. Specifier: Without accompanying intellectual impairment (IQ 90) but with significant variability between verbal and performance IQ, at risk for learning disability
3. Specifier: With fluid speech, but with pragmatic (social) language difficulty
4. Specifier: Associated with Fragile X syndrome. Complicating medical problem: sleep-onset disorder
5. Specifier: Associated with ADHD and anxiety as per evaluation from PCP, school educational specialists, and information provided by behavioral therapist

The recommended recording procedure for autism diagnosis offers an opportunity to clearly understand a child's strengths, weaknesses, and needs, and can help with guiding medical care in the PCP's office, support to families, and appropriate referrals. Based on the information gathered from the autism diagnostic team, the PCP office, the school, and the behavioral therapist, Caitlyn was identified in the school as having "Autism," which is one category under IDEA. An IEP was developed to meet Caitlyn's educational needs. Because of her difficulty with reading, Caitlyn received reading support in addition to social skills supports and visual supports to help with transitions. In the medical home, the PCP worked with the family to gather information regarding ADHD, and referred the family for behavioral therapy while waiting for the evaluation for possible autism. Although girls with Fragile X syndrome often have learning disability rather than intellectual disability, they often have the problems that Caitlyn presented with. The PCP referred the family to a Fragile X support group. Finally, this family benefited from ongoing support in the medical home. The PCP started melatonin for sleep-onset disorder. He also managed referrals and comanaged medication management for ADHD and anxiety with a psychiatrist the family saw twice a year. The family felt that their PCP was a true advocate for their child with ASD (**Box 7**).

Box 7
National Center for Medical Home Implementation

The National Center for Medical Home Implementation (NCMHI) is a cooperative agreement between the Maternal and Child Health Bureau (MCHB) and the American Academy of Pediatrics (AAP). The NCMHI is housed in the AAP Division of Children with Special Needs. Information specific to ASD is also available at http://www.aap.org/en-us/about-the-aap/ Committees-Councils-Sections/Council-on-Children-with-Disabilities/Pages/Recent-Information. aspx. At this Web site, AAP resources for professionals and families include:

- Sound Advice on Autism, which is a collection of interviews with pediatricians, researchers, and parents of children with ASD

- *Information on Autism: Caring for Children with Autism Spectrum Disorders: A Resources Toolkit for Clinicians*, second edition

- Information on the book: *Autism Spectrum Disorders: What Every Parent Needs to Know*

- Prevalence data from the CDC

- AAP policy documents related to ASD

REFERENCES

1. Centers for Disease Control and Prevention. In: Prevalence of Autism Spectrum Disorder Among Children Aged 8 Years: Autism and Developmental Disabilities Monitoring Network, 11 Sites, United States, 2010. Morbidity and Mortality Weekly Report 2014;63(SSo2):1–21.

2. American Psychiatric Association. Diagnostic and statistical manual of mental disorders. 5th edition. Washington, DC: American Psychiatric Association; 2013.

3. American Psychiatric Association. Diagnostic and statistical manual of mental disorders. 4th edition text revision. Washington, DC: American Psychiatric Association; 2000.

4. American Academy of Family Physicians. Patient-centered medical home. Available at: http://www.aafp.org/online/en/home/membership/initiatives/pcmh.html. Accessed August 4, 2010.

5. National Center for Medical Home Implementation. What is a family-centered medical home? Available at: http://www.medicalhomeinfo.org/. Accessed March 21, 2014.

6. Patient-Centered Primary Care Collaborative. Joint principles of the patient center medical home. Available at: http://www.pcpcc.net/content/joint-principles-patient-centered-medical-home. Accessed March 21, 2014.

7. Carbone P, Murphy N, Norlin C, et al. Parent and pediatrician perspectives regarding the primary care of children with autism spectrum disorder. J Autism Dev Disord 2013;43:964–72.

8. Myers SM, Johnson CP. Management of children with autism spectrum disorders. Pediatrics 2007;120:1162–82.

9. Golnik A, Ireland M, Borowsky IW. Medical homes for children with autism: a, physician survey. Pediatrics 2009;123:966–71.

10. Carbone PS, Behl DD, Azor V, et al. The medical home for children with autism spectrum disorders: parent and pediatrician perspectives. J Autism Dev Disord 2010;40:317–24.

11. Kogan MD, Strickland BB, Blumberg SJ, et al. A national profile of the health care experiences and family impact of autism spectrum disorder among children in the United States, 2005–2006. Pediatrics 2008;122:e1149–58.

12. Wiggins LD, Baio J, Rice C. Examination of the time between first evaluation and first autism spectrum diagnosis in a population-based sample. J Dev Behav Pediatr 2006;27:S79–87.

13. Carbone PS, Farley M, Davis T. Primary care for children with autism. Am Fam Physician 2010;8:453–60.

14. Howlin P, Asgharian A. The diagnosis of autism and Asperger syndrome: findings from a survey of 770 families. Dev Med Child Neurol 1999;41:834–9.

15. Sices L, Egbert L, Mercer MB. Sugar-coaters and straight talkers: communicating about developmental delays in primary care. Pediatrics 2009;124:e705–13.

16. Dawson G, Rogers S, Munson J, et al. Randomized, controlled trial of an intervention for toddlers with autism: the Early Start Denver Model. Pediatrics 2010;125:e17–23.

17. Child find. What is child find? 2010. Available at: http://www.childfindidea.org/. Accessed August 4, 2010.

18. Warren Z, Stone W, Humberd Q. A training model for the diagnosis of autism in community pediatric practice. J Dev Behav Pediatr 2009;30:442–6.

19. Johnson CP, Myers SM. Identification and evaluation of children with autism spectrum disorders. Pediatrics 2007;120:1183–215.

20. Norris M, Lecavalier L. Screening accuracy of level 2 autism spectrum disorder rating scales: a review of selected instruments. Autism 2010;14:263–84.

21. Klin A, Lang J, Cicchetti DV, et al. Brief report: interrater reliability of clinical diagnosis and DSM-IV criteria for autistic disorder: results of the DSM-IV autism field trial. J Autism Dev Disord 2000;30:163–7.

22. Ozonoff S, Dawson G, McParland J. A parent's guide to Asperger syndrome and high-functioning autism: how to meet the challenges and help your child thrive. New York: Guilford Press; 2002.

23. Rapin I, Tuchman RF. Autism: definition, neurobiology, screening, diagnosis. Pediatr Clin North Am 2008;55:1129–46, viii.

24. Huerta M, Lord C. Diagnostic evaluation of autism spectrum disorders. Pediatr Clin North Am 2012;59:103–11.

25. Aspy R, Grossman BG. The Ziggurat model. Shawnee Mission (KS): Autism Asperger Publishing Co; 2007.

26. Harrington J. Autism the school-aged child: diagnostic dilemma, comorbid condition, or both? Consultant for Pediatricians. 2013;12(1).

27. Levy SE, Giarelli E, Lee LC, et al. Autism spectrum disorder and co-occurring developmental, psychiatric, and medical conditions among children in multiple populations of the United States. J Dev Behav Pediatr 2010;31:267–75.

28. Simonoff E, Jones C, Pickles A, et al. Severe mood problems in adolescents with autism spectrum disorder. J Child Psychol Psychiatry 2012;53:1157–66.

29. Coury D. Medical treatment of autism spectrum disorders. Curr Opin Neurol 2010;23:131–6.

30. Buie T, Campbell DB, Fuchs GJ 3rd, et al. Evaluation, diagnosis, and treatment of gastrointestinal disorders in individuals with ASDs: a consensus report. Pediatrics 2010;125:S1–18.

31. Rhoades RA, Scarpa A, Salley B. The importance of physician knowledge of autism spectrum disorder: results of a parent survey. BMC Pediatr 2007;7:37.

32. Souders MC, Mason TB, Valladares O, et al. Sleep behaviors and sleep quality in children with autism spectrum disorders. Sleep 2009;32:1566–78.

33. Wright B, Sims D, Smart S, et al. Melatonin versus placebo in children with autism spectrum conditions and severe sleep problems not amenable to behaviour management strategies: a randomised controlled crossover trial. J Autism Dev Disord 2010;41:175–84.

34. Estes AM, Dawson G, Sterling L, et al. Level of intellectual functioning predicts patterns of associated symptoms in school-age children with autism spectrum disorder. Am J Ment Retard 2007;112:439–49.

35. Leyfer OT, Folstein SE, Bacalman S, et al. Comorbid psychiatric disorders in children with autism: interview development and rates of disorders. J Autism Dev Disord 2006;36:849–61.

36. Crosland KA, Zarcone JR, Lindauer SE, et al. Use of functional analysis methodology in the evaluation of medication effects. J Autism Dev Disord 2003;33: 271–9.

37. Green V, Pituch K, Itchon J, et al. Internet survey of treatments used by parents of children with autism. Res Dev Disabil 2006;27:70–84.

38. Reichow B. Overview of meta-analyses of early intensive behavioral intervention for young children with autism spectrum disorders. J Autism Dev Disord 2012;42: 512–20.

39. Simpson R. Evidence-based practices and students with autism spectrum disorders. Focus Autism Other Dev Disabil 2005;20:140–9.

40. Warren Z, McPheeters M, Sathe N, et al. A systematic review of early intensive intervention for autism spectrum disorders. Pediatrics 2011;127:1303–11.

41. Wink L, Erickson C, McDougle C. Pharmacologic treatment of behavioral symptoms associated with autism and other pervasive developmental disorders. Curr Treat Options Neurol 2010;12:529–38.

42. Hoekstra P, Troost P, Lahuis B, et al. Risperidone-induced weight gain in referred children with autism spectrum disorders is associated with a common polymorphism in the 5-hydroxtryptamine 2c receptor gene. J Child Adolesc Psychopharmacol 2010;20:473–7.

43. McDougle CJ, Scahill L, Aman MG, et al. Risperidone for the core symptom domains of autism: results from the study by the autism network of the research units on pediatric psychopharmacology. Am J Psychiatry 2005;162: 1142–8.

44. Mandell D, Novak M, Zubritsky C. Factors associated with age of diagnosis among children with autism spectrum disorders. Pediatrics 2005;116:1480–6.

45. Grinker RR. Unstrange minds: remapping the world of autism. Philadelphia: Basic Books; 2007.

46. Flanagan-Klygis EA, Sharp L, Frader JE. Dismissing the family who refuses vaccines: a study of pediatrician attitudes. Arch Pediatr Adolesc Med 2005; 159:929–34.

47. Halperin B, Melnychuk R, Downie J, et al. When is it permissible to dismiss a family who refuses vaccines? Legal, ethical and public health perspectives. Paediatr Child Health 2007;12:843–5.

48. Liptak GS, Orlando M, Yingling JT, et al. Satisfaction with primary health care received by families of children with developmental disabilities. J Pediatr Health Care 2006;20:245–52.

49. Levy SE, Hyman SL. Complementary and alternative medicine treatments for children with autism spectrum disorders. Child Adolesc Psychiatr Clin N Am 2008;17:803–20, ix.

50. American Academy of Pediatrics. Children's health topics: autism: American Academy of Pediatrics. Available at: http://www.aap.org/healthtopics/autism.cfm. Accessed August 4, 2010.

51. Centers for Disease Control and Prevention. Learn the signs. Act early. Available at: http://www.cdc.gov/ncbddd/actearly/index.html. Accessed August 4, 2010.

Managing Attention-Deficit/Hyperactivity Disorder in Children and Adolescents

Elizabeth K. McClain, PhD, EdS, MPH[a],*, Erin Jewell Burks, DO[b]

KEYWORDS

- Attention-deficit/hyperactivity disorder • DSM-V • Pharmacologic approaches
- Nonpharmacologic approaches • Shared decision making • Stimulant medication
- Nonstimulant medication • Adolescents

KEY POINTS

- 6.4 million children aged 4–17 are diagnosed with ADHD, but only 3.5 million reported taking medication for ADHD.
- Updates in the DSM-V diagnostic criteria for ADHD including age ranges and environment sare discussed.
- Pharmacologic therapy serves as front line treatment for ADHD including both stimulant and non-stimulant therapy.
- Medical management of side effects is a key factor in adherence to treatment.
- Non-pharmacologic approaches such as behavioral and cognitive therapies can provide an effective alternative for treatment of ADHD Adolescent views of ADHD differ from adults and share decision making and self management strategies can improv adherence to treatment.
- Teens with ADHD may be at a increased risks of substance abuse, but several intervention strategies have demonstrated effectiveness for early intervention. Educational resources to support ADHD are available through the Individuals with Disabilities Act and Americans with Disabilities Act Section 504.

BACKGROUND

Attention-deficit/hyperactivity disorder (ADHD) is the most frequently diagnosed neurodevelopmental disorder.[1,2] The percentage of children between 4 and 17 years of age diagnosed with ADHD has consistently increased in less than a decade from

[a] Department of Primary Care Medicine, Kansas City University of Medicine and Biosciences College of Osteopathic Medicine, 1750 Independence Avenue, Kansas City, MO 64106, USA; [b] Department of Psychiatry, School of Medicine, University of Missouri-Kansas City, 1000 E. 24th Street, Kansas City, MO 64108, USA
* Corresponding author.
E-mail address: emcclain@kcumb.edu

Prim Care Clin Office Pract 42 (2015) 99–112
http://dx.doi.org/10.1016/j.pop.2014.09.014   **primarycare.theclinics.com**

7.8% in 2003 to 9.5% in 2007.[1] As of 2011, 11.0% (6.4 million) have been diagnosed with ADHD.[1] Sex differences have also been identified, with boys (13.2%) more likely to obtain a diagnosis when compared with girls (5.6%).[1] When comparing 2003 to 2011, these data indicate that the proportion of children having a history of ADHD has increased by 42% in less than a decade. This finding translates to an estimated increase of 2 million additional children/adolescents aged 4 to 17 years diagnosed with ADHD in 2011 in the United States alone. Adolescents with ADHD are much less willing to pursue or adhere to medication or psychosocial therapy often because their perceptions of side effects or perceived value of treatment. Adolescents with ADHD, therefore, experience an increased risk for challenges because of performance issues at school, work, and home environments These adolescents often demonstrated an inability to meet common expectations for increased independence in organization, time management, and schoolwork without continued formal ADHD treatment. According to a parent report, more than 3.5 million children in the United States, or 6% of 4 to 17 year olds, were reported by their parents to be taking medication for ADHD, marking a 28% increase from 2007–2008 to 2011–2012.[1] According to data reports there is variation on adherence to ADHD prescribed treatments including medication and mental health therapy. Reports show that approximately 7 out of 10 children or (69%) of children with current ADHD diagnosis report current medication therapy.[1] Whereas only 5 out of 10 children or (51%) report ongoing treatment or counseling from a mental health professional.[1] Finally when all data is combined, 8 out of 10 children or 82.5% of children diagnosed with ADHD currently receive either medication or ongoing mental health treatment for their ADHD diagnosis.[1]

DEFINITION

ADHD is characterized by a pattern of behavior that must be present in multiple settings, such as work, school, or home. This pattern of behavior can negatively impact performance across multiple environments, including social, education, or work. Symptoms are divided into 3 categories: (1) inattention, (2) hyperactivity and impulsivity, and (3) combined (if criteria for both inattention and hyperactivity and impulsivity are met). The standard accepted diagnostic criteria for ADHD diagnosis is provided through the American Psychiatric Association's *Diagnostic and Statistical Manual of Mental Disorders*.[3] The fifth edition (*DSM-V*) was released in May 2013 replacing the fourth edition. The Centers for Disease Control and Prevention has focused on the use of a common standard of diagnosis across communities in an effort to improve accuracy in determining the number of children diagnosed with ADHD and the public health impact this condition has across communities.

CHANGES FROM THE *DIAGNOSTIC AND STATISTICAL MANUAL OF MENTAL DISORDERS* (FOURTH EDITION) TO THE *DIAGNOSTIC AND STATISTICAL MANUAL OF MENTAL DISORDERS* (FIFTH EDITION) CRITERIA

The following specific changes were made in the *DSM-5* for the diagnosis of ADHD[3] (see http://www.cdc.gov/ncbddd/adhd/diagnosis.html):

- Symptoms can occur by 12 years of age rather than by 6 years of age.
- Several symptoms are required to be present in multiple settings rather than just some impairment in more than one setting.
- Descriptions of symptoms now include examples for older ages (17 years of age to adult).
- Older adolescents and adults must exhibit 5 instead of 6 of the criteria.

PHARMACOLOGIC STRATEGIES

Pharmacotherapy is an important component in the treatment and management of symptoms associated with ADHD. Stimulants are the first approach to effective treatment of hyperactivity and disruptive behaviors, and clinical studies suggest a patient success response rate of 70% to 80%.[4]

- *Stimulant therapy* is used to treat both moderate and severe ADHD and can increase alertness, attention, and energy in addition to elevating blood pressure (BP), heart rate, and respiration. Studies have reported parental difference in use of medication for their children that is dependent on the child's ADHD subtype diagnosis (**Fig. 1**). This medication therapy may help children and adolescents focus their thoughts and ignore distractions to increase success across settings including school, work, and home. The most commonly used stimulant medications are methylphenidate (MPH) and amphetamines. Evidence demonstrates that these stimulants are safe when prescribed to healthy children monitored under medical supervision (**Table 1**).[5]
- *Nonstimulant therapy* is another option to treat ADHD. Approximately 30% of patients fail to respond to stimulant therapy and need to pursue other treatment options.[4] Nonstimulant therapy is often chosen as an alternative if stimulant therapy is ineffective, if children experience side effects associated with taking stimulant medications, or if children have other conditions along with ADHD. There are 3 nonstimulant medications approved by the Food and Drug Administration (FDA) for use in children diagnosed with ADHD to help reduce symptoms. Both extended-release (XR) guanfacine (Intuniv) and XR clonidine (Kapvay) are also FDA approved to be used in combination with stimulant treatment to increase the reduction of ADHD symptoms. This treatment combination may be preferred when stimulants are working, but additional reduction of symptoms is warranted. The third medication is atomoxetine (ATX; Strattera). It is not yet FDA approved for combination therapy; it is sometimes used in in addition to current stimulants as an off-label combination therapy (**Table 2**).

MRI EFFECTS OF STIMULANT MEDICATION

Stimulant medication treatment of ADHD has been proven effective. However, concerns remain regarding the physiologic longitudinal impact of medication on the

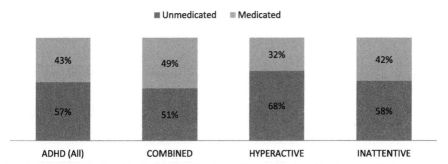

Fig. 1. Percentage of children diagnosed with ADHD taking medication by ADHD subtype. (*Data from* Substance Abuse and Mental Health Services Administration. Shared decision-making in mental health care: practice, research, and future directions. HHS Publication No. SMA-09-4371. Rockville (MD): Center for Mental Health Services; Substance Abuse and Mental Health Services Administration; 2010.)

Table 1
FDA-approved ADHD stimulant medication

Class	Trade/Brand Name	Generic Medication Name	Frequency
Amphetamines	Adderall	Mixed amphetamine salts	QD-BID
	Adderall XR	Extended-release mixed amphetamine salts	QD
	Dexedrine	Dextroamphetamine	BID-TID
	Dexedrine Spansule	Dextroamphetamine	QD-BID
	Vyvanse	Lisdexamfetamine (extended release)	QD
MPH	Concerta	MPH	QD
	Daytrana	MPH (patch)	Apply for 9 h
	Focalin	Dexmethylphenidate	BID
	Focalin XR	Extended-release dexmethylphenidate	QD
	Metadate ER	Extended-release MPH	QD
	Metadate CD	Extended-release MPH	QD
	Methylin	MPH hydrochloride (liquid & chewable tablets)	BID-TID
	Quillivant XR	Extended release MPH (liquid)	QD
	Ritalin	MPH	BID-TID
	Ritalin LA	Extended-release MPH	QD
	Ritalin SR	Extended-release MPH	QD-BID

Abbreviations: BID, twice daily; FDA, Food and Drug Administration; QD, daily; TID, 3 times daily.
From American Academy of Child & Adolescent Psychiatry and American Psychiatric Association. ADHD parents medication guide. Available at: https://www.aacap.org/App_Themes/AACAP/Docs/resource_centers/adhd/adhd_parents_medication_guide_201305.pdf. Accessed March 4, 2014; with permission.

developing brain.[6] Research has used MRIs to study changes in the brain and identify the physiologic impact of medication on children with ADHD. These studies found that the MRI results of individuals with ADHD taking therapeutic doses of stimulants were more similar to non-ADHD individual controls than to nonmedicated individuals with ADHD individuals. These findings were supported by the consistent direction of all structural and connectivity findings, and nearly all functional activation findings, which included brain measures in medicated groups of persons with ADHD compared with both control groups and nonmedicated ADHD groups.[6–8]

Clinical Implications

Evidence from multiple MRI studies indicates that concerns regarding the negative impact of stimulant medication are unfounded and that treatment with stimulants should be considered if appropriate for the clinical presentation of patients.[6–8]

Table 2
FDA-approved ADHD nonstimulant medication

Class	Trade Name	Generic Name	
Norepinephrine uptake inhibitor	Strattera	Atomoxetine	QD-BID
	Intuniv[a]	XR guanfacine	QD
Alpha adrenergic agents	Kapvay[a]	XR clonidine	QD-BID

Abbreviations: QD, daily; BID, twice daily; TID, 3 times daily.
[a] FDA approved to be added to stimulant treatment to reduce ADHD symptoms.
Data from American Academy of Child & Adolescent Psychiatry and American Psychiatric Association. ADHD Parents Medication Guide. Available at: https://www.aacap.org/App_Themes/AACAP/Docs/resource_centers/adhd/adhd_parents_medication_guide_201305.pdf. Accessed March 4, 2014.

- Results also increase the possibility that brain changes associated with stimulant treatment might account for stimulant-associated improvements in neuro-cognition and other areas.[6-8]
- Of particular interest is the possibility that, given the wide range of brain areas affected, stimulants could improve several neurocognitive functions.
- Stimulant medication is associated with the reduction of ADHD-associated brain abnormalities or the normalization of basal ganglia abnormalities in ADHD.[6-8]

MANAGEMENT OF SIDE EFFECTS

Side effects are common experiences for many children treated with ADHD medication. The most frequently noted side effects from stimulant medication include appetite reduction, weight loss, sleep disturbance, headaches, and stomach pain. Less common side effects include delayed growth in height. This delay often occurs during the first 2 years of treatment, with the growth rate returning to normal in the following years.[9] Infrequently, underlying mood and anxiety disorders, depression, psychosis, or suicidal ideation may increase with ADHD medication. It is important for physicians to work with patients and families to educate, identify, and manage side effects to facilitate the effectiveness and adherence to ADHD therapy.

LOSS OF APPETITE AND GROWTH DELAY

Both stimulant and nonstimulant medications, MPH and ATX, are associated with a loss of appetite in the short term.[10] Stimulants and ATX may be associated with delays in height and weight gain.[11]

Further evidence is needed on the effect on appetite loss in the midterm and long-term and to identify if there are significant differences in appetite reduction among different drug classes, formulations, and doses. Growth delays are dose dependent but reversible after treatment cessation.[10]

Management of Appetite Loss and Growth Delay

- There should be 6-month interval assessments of appetite, weight, height, and body mass index.
- Identify any pretreatment eating concerns and monitor them separately from medication-induced variations in eating.[11]
- Medication should be taken following meals not before meals.
- Consume calorie-dense healthy snacks and late-evening snacks.
- Reduce the dose or select an alternative drug class.[11]
- Incorporate drug holidays or scheduled breaks in medication therapy to provide a window for growth catch up.[10,11]
- Consult a pediatric endocrinologist for significant concerns with height, weight, and growth values less than the critical thresholds.[11]

CARDIOVASCULAR CONCERNS

Stimulant and nonstimulant (ATX) medications have been associated with small increases in blood pressure (BP) (mean systolic BP and diastolic BP) and heart rate that are time limited and linked to treatment.[10] A small percentage of individuals (5%-15%) may present with increases to more than the 95th percentile in BP.[12] There is no evidence supporting that stimulant or nonstimulant medications are associated with significant changes in electrocardiographic values.[13] Guanfacine- XR or clonidine-XR may be associated with minor decreases in BP (mean systolic BP and diastolic BP) and heart rate mean systolic BP, diastolic BP, and heart rate when they are administered alone or in combination with stimulant medication.[11] There is no evidence to support a significant association between stimulant or nonstimulant medications and severe cardiovascular events (sudden cardiac death, acute myocardial infarction, and stroke).[12]

Cardiac Issues Before Initiating Attention-Deficit/Hyperactivity Disorder Medication and Medication Management

- Complete a clinical interview to identify a cardiovascular risk factor.
- Establish a baseline heart rate and BP.
- Monitor the heart rate at 3- to 6-month intervals once medication therapy is initiated.
- Perform an auscultation to detect any murmurs and make appropriate referrals as indicated.
- A systematic electrocardiogram is not mandatory and should only be conducted when specifically indicated.

SLEEP DISTURBANCE

Sleep disturbance may be associated with the use of ADHD medications.[10] However, often children with ADHD experience sleep disturbances that are not linked to medication. Therefore, it is importance to assess the nature of sleep disturbances as well as the relationship to other variables, including medication.[14] Completion of an objective assessment of sleep with polysomnography is indicated if there are concerns of sleep-breathing disorder, episodic nocturnal phenomena, limb movements, and unexplained excessive daytime sleepiness. There is no extensive evidence for differential effects on sleep of different medication classes or formulations. Stimulants may increase patterns of reduced sleep and delayed sleep onset, whereas nonstimulants may increase fatigue and patterns of increased sleep.

Management of Sleep Problems with Behavioral Interventions

- Monitor current sleep and implement sleep hygiene.
- Clinical interview or sleep questionnaires and sleep diaries are suggested to screen and monitor sleep disturbances.
- Consider stopping the current medication if it is possible.
- Consider assessing for stress and anxiety.

If Behavioral Interventions Are Not Effective

- Assess for and treat restless leg syndrome.[10]
- Assess for the rebound effect with psychostimulants, and consider the addition of smaller doses of short-acting psychostimulants in the evening.

If Psychostimulant Is the Current Treatment

- Consider dose reduction, alternative classes or formulations of stimulants, or the use of nonstimulant medications.[10]
- Consider adding melatonin.

TICS

ADHD is the most common comorbid diagnosis for individuals with Tourette syndrome, with a 60% to 80% patient report in clinical samples.[10,13] It has also been determined that stimulant medication MPH and dextroamphetamine may worsen tics. Comorbid tic symptoms may significantly decrease with nonstimulant medication (ATX).

Management of Tics

- Monitor tic intensity and frequency over 3 months before making a decision regarding the ADHD treatment protocol.
- Reduce the dosage of the current medication and monitor for reduction or elimination of tics.
- Substitute the medication class or formulation.
- An alpha-2-agonist (guanfacine) may be an effective option targeting ADHD behaviors and tic reduction.[15]
- Use of a norepinephrine reuptake inhibitor (ATX) has also been effective with ADHD as well as tic reduction.[15]
- If the dose reduction or substitution prove to be ineffective, the addition of an antipsychotic (tiapride, sulpiride, or clonidine) can be used to control tics

MEDICATION MISUSE/ABUSE

There is no evidence that treatment with a stimulant or nonstimulant medication increases the risk for later substance use disorders (SUD).[10] No differences in substance abuse rates were reported for children currently using ADHD medication compared with children with ADHD who were no longer taking ADHD medication. However, adolescents with ADHD have demonstrated an increased risk of substance abuse when compared with non-ADHD peers.[11]

- Daily cigarette smoking was reported with 17% of the adolescents with ADHD compared with 8% of non-ADHD teens.[16]
- Alcohol use was high in both groups, highlighting its common occurrence for teenagers in general.[16]
- At 15 years of age, 35% of those with ADHD histories reported using one or more substances as compared with only 20% of teens without ADHD histories.[16]
- Ten percent of adolescents with ADHD met the criteria for an SUD or dependence disorder, which means they experienced significant problems from their substance use as compared with only 3% of the non-ADHD group.[16]
- At 17 years of age, marijuana abuse or dependence was reported to be 13% versus 7% of the ADHD and non-ADHD groups, respectively.[16]

Management of Misuse and Abuse

- In patients with ADHD who also exhibit signs of or are diagnosed with SUD, the treatment of SUD needs to be addressed first, with ADHD treatment quickly following.
- If patients have current or previous documented substance abuse, it is important to closely monitor the use of prescribed stimulants.
- In high-risk cases, an XR formulation of a stimulant or the use of a nonstimulant is recommended.
- The addition of intensive behavior therapy, with or without medication management, was less likely to initiate substance use in early adolescence.[17,18]

Management of Seizures

In patients with well-controlled epilepsy, stimulants (MPH) were associated with a low risk for seizure.[10] For nonstimulants (ATX), both efficacy and short-term safety have yet to be established.

- Electroencephalographic screening is not currently indicated for patients with ADHD without a history of seizures.

- The management of ADHD in children with epilepsy includes specific pharmaco-therapy for ADHD.
- Nonspecific interventions include decreasing antiepileptic polypharmacy, reducing drug interactions, and switching to antiepileptic drugs with fewer cognitive and behavioral effects.[17,18]

RARELY OCCURRING SYMPTOMS (PSYCHOSIS AND SUICIDAL IDEATION)

Psychotic symptoms or suicidal thoughts and behaviors rarely occur during treatment with ADHD drugs.[10] Children with ADHD often have other psychiatric disorders, with epidemiologic studies suggesting comorbidity rates between 50% and 90%.[1] High rates of psychiatric comorbidity have been reported both in psychiatric and pediatric patient populations. Therefore, it is important to identify risk factors and assess behavioral symptoms and psychiatric concerns with variables, including medication.[14] The completion of a behavioral screening assessment with psychiatric or psychological consult is suggested (**Figs. 2** and **3**).

Management of Rarely Occurring Symptoms

Psychotic symptoms

- The reduction or discontinuation of medication is an appropriate course of action.[10]
- Following the resolution of the symptoms, ADHD medication can be reintroduced with close monitoring.

Suicidal thoughts and behaviors

- An initial formal standardized screening tool should be used during the assessment or initial treatment.[10] If there are concerns, a formal suicide rating scale should be administered.
- Refer to a mental health specialist to diagnosis and assist with the management of a psychiatric disorder.
- If severe suicidal thoughts and behaviors are documented, the reduction or discontinuation of medication is recommended (though there is no contraindication for ADHD medication).

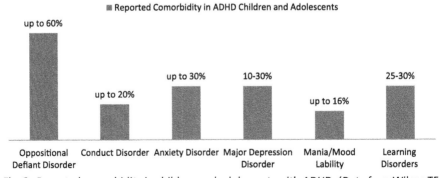

Fig. 2. Reported comorbidity in children and adolescents with ADHD. (*Data from* Wilens TE, Biederman J, Brown S, et al. Psychiatric comorbidity and functioning in clinically referred preschool children and school-age youths with ADHD. J Am Acad Child Adolesc Psychiatry 2002;41:262–8; and Visser SN, Cuffe SP, Holbrook JR, et al. Patterns in ADHD medication use among an epidemiologic cohort of youth. Poster presented at AACAP, Toronto (Canada). 2010. (As cited in PLAY study findings [Project to Learn About ADHD in Youth] CDC Web site). Available at: http://www.cdc.gov/ncbddd/adhd/play2.html. Accessed March 13, 2014.)

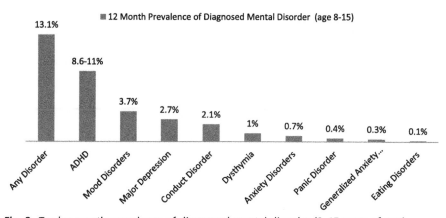

Fig. 3. Twelve-month prevalence of diagnosed mental disorder (8–15 years of age).

NONPHARMACOLOGIC STRATEGIES
Psychosocial Treatments

Therapeutic interventions, such as behavioral and cognitive therapies, provide another approach in the treatment of ADHD. These therapies focus on reducing ADHD-related behaviors through reinforcement of desired behaviors. They focus on instilling positive habits that increase functioning and success at home, at school, and in social relationships. Psychosocial treatments are not as effective as medicine for treating the core symptoms of ADHD. However, they are another treatment option to complement medication therapy and can serve as an option for adolescents and parents who do not want to use medication (**Table 3**).

Resources

- CHADD (Child and Adults with Attention Deficit Disorders) psychosocial resources
- Parent training, health: children.org
- American Academy of Child and Adolescent Psychiatry: ADHD resources
- Clinical guidelines from the National Institute for Health Care and Clinical Excellence
- http://www.nice.org.uk/nicemedia/live/12061/42059/42059.pdf

EDUCATIONAL SUPPORTS

It is important for the primary care physician to be aware of educational services available for children, adolescents, and young adults with ADHD. This awareness can increase physician communication regarding treatment or behavioral programs in the home, school, and other settings, such as recreational or work environments. Children and adolescents with a diagnosis of ADHD can benefit from formal and informal school supports. However, parents may not be aware of services available or may not know how to pursue eligibility for services. Additional challenges for parents may include variability in eligibility criteria or service delivery by state as well as by school district. Children can formally be referred through the public school district for a psychoeducational evaluation with a multidisciplinary team. Following an evaluation qualification, special education services or regular education services are determined. Children with ADHD can qualify for an individual education plan under "other health impairment classification" through the Individuals with Disabilities Act (IDEA)

Table 3
Levels of evidence-based behavioral treatments for ADHD descriptions and outcomes

Treatment Type	Outcomes
Considered well-established treatments	
BPT Behavior-modification principles are provided to parents for implementation in home settings.	• Increased student compliance with parental commands • Increased parental understanding of behavioral principles • High report of parental satisfaction
Behavioral classroom management Behavior-modification principles are provided to teachers for implementation in classroom settings.	• Increased student attention to instruction and improved work productivity • Increased student compliance with classroom rules • Reduced student disruptive behavior
BPI Interventions are focused on peer interactions/relationships; these are often group-based interventions provided weekly and include clinic-based social-skills training used either alone or concurrently with behavioral parent training and/or medication.	• Minimal effects from office-based interventions • Minimal positive effects on parent ratings of ADHD symptoms found by studies of BPI combined with clinic-based BPT • Some concern with social validity of interventions
Organizational skills training Out-of-school or in-class sessions are focused on organization, time management, and planning skills. Interventions can be individual or peer-group based.	• Improvements of organization of materials • Improvement of homework management • Improvement of time management and planning
Considered possibly efficacious	
Neurofeedback training EEG neurofeedback focuses on the central nervous system and the brain's activity in order to give moment-to-moment information. Children with ADHD have higher rates of EEG abnormalities compared with children without ADHD, such as higher theta wave rhythms (drowsiness), lower sensorimotor rhythms (movement control), and lower beta waves (attention and memory processes). Neurofeedback provides audio and visual interpretations of these brain waves, and children learn how to maintain the appropriate levels for functioning.	• Concerns with efficacy caused by methodological issues and data reporting • Improved regulated cortical activity associated with clinical improvement • Improvement in preparation and increased allocation of attention to objective tests of attention • NF training superior to a computerized AST • Behavioral improvements from NF training in children with ADHD maintained at 6-mo follow-up

Abbreviations: AST, attention skills training; BPI, behavioral peer interventions; BPT, behavioral parent training; EEG, electroencephalogram; NF, neurofeedback.

Data from Pelham W, Fabiano GA. Evidence-based psychosocial treatments for attention-deficit/hyperactivity disorder. J Clin Child Adolesc Psychol 2008;37(1):184–214; and Evans SW, Sarno Owens J, Bunford N. Evidence-based psychosocial treatments for children and adolescents with attention-deficit hyperactivity disorder. J Clin Child Adolesc Psychol 2014;43:527–51.

Box 1
Examples of resources and testing accommodations

Educational Testing Systems: https://www.ets.org/disabilities/documentation/documenting_adhd/

Scholastic Aptitude Test: http://sat.collegeboard.org/register/for-students-with-disabilities

American College Testing: http://www.actstudent.org/regist/disab/

College Board Services: www.collegeboard.com/ssd/student

United States Medical Licensing Examination: http://www.usmle.org/test-accommodations/

Comprehensive Osteopathic Medical Licensing Examination: http://www.nbome.org/candidates.asp?m=can

IDEA: http://idea.ed.gov/

Americans with Disability Act Section 504: http://www.ada.gov/

---

and receive services through special education. Services can also be obtained through regular education with the 504 Rehabilitation Act. A behavioral plan can be developed through regular education funding. Both plans can provide additional supports, such as classroom adaptions, behavioral systems, modified work assignments, or testing arrangements. These supports can extend to college and graduate studies, including testing modifications for national high-stakes examinations (**Box 1**).

Shared Decision Making

Shared decision making (SDM) is a strategy that is used to match patients and families with the most acceptable approaches to treatments. In SDM, both clinicians and

---

Box 2
Steps for shared decision-making

- Invite patients to participate
  - Recognition that a decision needs to be made
  - Identification of partners in the process as equals
- Present the options and state the options as equal
  - Provide information on benefit and risk
- Assist patients in evaluating options based on their goals/concerns
  - Shared exploration of understanding and expectations
  - Identifying preferences
- Facilitate deliberation and decision making
  - Negotiating options/concordance
  - Sharing the decision
- Assist with implementation
  - Arranging follow-up to evaluate decision-making outcomes

Adapted from Substance Abuse and Mental Health Services Administration. Shared decision-making in mental health care: practice, research, and future directions. HHS Publication No.SMA-09-4371. Rockville (MD): Center for Mental Health Services; Substance Abuse and Mental Health Services Administration; 2010.

families participate in treatment decisions, exchange information, express preferences, and jointly determine a treatment plan. For this process to be effective, physicians, parents, and adolescents must have a shared understanding of other perspectives. This shared understanding includes the ADHD condition and its treatment as well as the health and health history of the patients. Effective SDM approaches incorporate all strategies stated above. As a result, decisions reflect the collective needs, preferences, and goals balanced with the appropriate scientific evidence (**Box 2**).

Self-Management Strategies

Adherence attitudes
Adolescents' views regarding their willingness to seek ADHD treatment differs significantly from the adults who are also involved their treatment process.[2]

- Overall, adolescents with ADHD expressed less willingness to use pharmacologic or psychosocial therapy for ADHD when compared with parents and health professionals.
- For adolescents, a willingness to use pharmacologic or psychosocial therapy increased when they felt knowledgeable or thought the treatment therapy was effective and acceptable.
- However, adolescents' willingness to use pharmacologic or psychosocial therapy decreased if they anticipated negative side effects.

Box 3
Adolescent transition to autonomy in perception of ADHD treatment and adherence

Adolescent self-appraisal of functional impact of ADHD and/or medication

- Impact at school
- Social impact
- Impact of stigma
- Impact on creativity
- Impact on driving skills

Adolescent involvement in discussions and decision making that were perceived to increase over time

- Silent bystander
- Ambivalent reporter
- Active reporter
- Contributor to dosage adjustments
- Gaining a voice
- Vocal protester not given a vote
- Parent supervision of medication taking
- Covert medication disposal
- Overt trials on and off medication

Adolescent movement to full autonomy in medication management

- Selective use depending on perceived need to successfully complete tasks (tests, sports)
- Future medicine use depended on primary perceived purpose of medication (academics)
- Trade-offs

Implications for clinical practice

- It is important for primary care physicians to gain a deeper understanding of the factors that contribute to adolescent medication treatment decisions to better facilitate clinician and family efforts to optimize adherence management of ADHD in adolescents (**Box 3**).[19]
- Medical professionals incorporated adolescents and made them feel part of SDM, and collaborative care processes were viewed in a more positive regard.[2]
- The most common descriptions of positive medical provider interactions by both parents and adolescents included specific mentions of active listening skills, such as good eye contact.

Medical professional expertise was important, but the manner in which the practitioner answered questions and focused on health literacy and education were more important to parents and adolescents.[19]

- Adolescents assume an increasing role in managing medication for ADHD but may benefit from support.
- Well-structured and coordinated trials where medication is stopped and outcomes relevant to adolescents, parents, teachers and/or doctors are measured, may help ensure a developmentally appropriate transition from family to self-management of ADHD.

SUMMARY

Almost half of children and adolescents are expected to require treatment of ADHD in adulthood, which, according the data released in 2011, may equate to 3.2 million adults.[20]

Those at greatest risk will be individuals with coexisting disruptive disorders, anxiety, smoking, and substance abuse. Early diagnosis and treatment that continues through transitions to adolescence are vital to facilitate continued success. Practitioners can incorporate both medication and behavioral therapy; using SDM can help these individuals develop autonomy and self-management strategies to manage their symptoms and succeed in adulthood.

REFERENCES

1. Centers for Disease Control and Prevention. Mental health surveillance among children — United States 2005–2011. MMWR Surveill Summ 2013;62(Suppl 2):1–35.
2. Busing R, Koro-Ljungbert M, Noguci K, et al. Willingness to use ADHD treatments: a mixed methods study of perceptions by adolescents, parents, health professionals and teachers. Soc Sci Med 2012;74:92–100.
3. American Psychiatric Association. Diagnostic and statistical manual of mental disorders. 5th edition. Arlington (VA): American Psychiatric Association; 2013.
4. van de Weijer-Bergsma E, Formsma AR, de Bruin EI, et al. The effectiveness of mindfulness training on behavioral problems and attentional functioning in adolescents with ADHD. J Child Fam Stud 2012;21:775–87.
5. Pliszka S. Psychostimulants. In: Rosenburg D, Gershon S, editors. Pharmacotherapy of child and adolescent psychiatric disorders. 3rd edition. Hoboken (NJ): Wiley-Blackwell; 2012. p. 65–104.
6. Spencer TJ, Brown A, Seidma LJ, et al. Effect of psychostimulants on brain structure and function in ADHD: a qualitative literature review of magnetic resonance imaging-based neuroimaging studies. J Clin Psychiatry 2013;74:902–17.

7. Nakao T, Radua J, Rubia K, et al. Gray matter volume abnormalities in ADHD: voxel-based meta-analysis exploring the effects of age and stimulant medication. Am J Psychiatry 2011;168(11):1154–63.

8. Frodl T, Skokauskas N. Meta-analysis of structural MRI studies in children and adults with attention deficit hyperactivity disorder indicates treatment effects. Acta Psychiatr Scand 2012;125(2):114–26. http://dx.doi.org/10.1/j.160-047. 2011.01786.x.

9. Faraone SV, Biederman J, Morley CP, et al. Effect of stimulants on height and weight: a review of the literature. J Am Acad Child Adolesc Psychiatry 2008; 47(9):994–1009.

10. Samuele Cortese S, Holtmann M, Banaschewski T, et al. Practitioner review: current best practice in the management of adverse events during treatment with ADHD medications in children and adolescents. J Child Psychol Psychiatry 2013;54(3):227–46.

11. Martinez-Raga J, Knecht C, Szeman N, et al. Risk of serious cardiovascular problems with medications for attention-deficit hyperactivity disorder. CNS Drugs 2013;27(1):15–30.

12. Konofala E, Lecendreuxa M, Cortesec S. Sleep and ADHD. Sleep Med 2010; 11(7):652–8.

13. Allen AJ, Kurlan RM, Gilbert DL, et al. Atomoxetine treatment in children and adolescents with ADHD and comorbid tic disorders. Neurology 2005;65:1941–9.

14. Rizzo R, Guilsano M. Chapter fourteen – clinical pharmacology of comorbid attention deficit hyperactivity disorder in Tourette syndrome. Advances in the neurochemistry and neuropharmacology of Tourette syndrome. Int Rev Neurobiol 2013;112:415–44.

15. Molina B, Hinshaw SP, Arnold LE, et al. Adolescent substance use in the multimodal treatment study of attention-deficit/hyperactivity disorder (ADHD) (MTA) as a function of childhood ADHD, random assignment to childhood treatments, and subsequent medication. J Am Acad Child Adolesc Psychiatry 2013;52:250–63.

16. Molina BS, Pelham WE, Gnagy EM, et al. Attention-deficit/hyperactivity disorder risk for heavy drinking and alcohol use disorder is age-specific. Alcohol Clin Exp Res 2007;31(4):643–54.

17. Slesnick N, Kaminer Y, Kelly J. Most common psychosocial interventions for adolescent substance use disorders. In: Kaminer Y, Bukstein OG, editors. Adolescent substance abuse. Psychiatric comorbidity and high-risk behaviors. New York: Routledge, Taylor & Francis Group; 2008. p. 111–44.

18. Brinkman WB, Sherman SN, Zmitrovich AR, et al. In their own words: adolescent views on ADHD and their evolving role managing medication. Acad Pediatr 2012; 12(1):57–61.

19. Spencer T, Biederman J, Wilens T. Attention-deficit/hyperactivity disorder and comorbidity. Pediatr Clin North Am 1999;46:915–27, vii.

20. Biederman J, Monuteaux MC, Spencer T, et al. Stimulant therapy and risk for subsequent substance use disorders in male adults with ADHD: a naturalistic controlled 10-year follow-up study. Am J Psychiatry 2008;165(5):597–603.

Food and Environmental Allergies

Miranda M. Huffman, MD, MEd

KEYWORDS

- Food allergies • Environmental allergies • IgE-mediated reactions • Atopic disease
- Immunotherapy

KEY POINTS

- Environmental allergies cause nasal and ophthalmologic symptoms that can be debilitating in themselves and exacerbate symptoms of asthma.
- Food allergies can cause a wide range of symptoms, from mild rashes to anaphylaxis. Although the exact incidence is hard to determine, it is likely increasing.
- Food allergies require an accurate diagnosis based on a combination of a comprehensive history and use of either skin-prick testing or food-specific serum immunoglobulin E levels.
- Environmental allergies should be treated with pharmacologic measures and avoidance strategies, with immunotherapy if needed.
- Food allergies should be treated with strict avoidance, and physicians should ensure that patients and their families have access to an autoinjector of epinephrine to keep on hand at all times in case of accidental exposure.

INTRODUCTION
Nature of the Problem

Allergic reactions to substances in our environment, including food, are important disease entities in and of themselves, in addition to their ability to exacerbate other chronic medical conditions such as asthma and eczema.

The incidence of allergic disease is difficult to ascertain, as there is great variance from study to study, and self-reported allergies are much more common than clinically confirmed allergies.[1] Frequency of disease varies based on location, but in the United States:

- Approximately 10% of individuals younger than 17 years had hay fever in the last year[2]
- Approximately 8% of children ages 6 to 18 years have a food allergy[3]

Department of Community and Family Medicine, University of Missouri-Kansas City, 2301 Charlotte Street, Kansas City, MO 64108, USA
E-mail address: Miranda.huffman@tmcmed.org

Prim Care Clin Office Pract 42 (2015) 113–128
http://dx.doi.org/10.1016/j.pop.2014.09.010
0095-4543/15/$ – see front matter © 2015 Elsevier Inc. All rights reserved.

Disease rates of environmental allergies appear to have stabilized[4] after a decade of increasing. However, the incidence of food allergies appears to be increasing.[5,6] Most children will eventually outgrow allergies to milk, soy, wheat, and egg; peanut and tree-nut allergies are more likely to persist into adulthood.[7] Seafood (including shellfish) allergies are more common in adults than in children.[7]

> Milk, eggs, and peanuts are the most common food allergens in the United States.[1]

Symptoms of allergic disease can affect nearly any system in the body (see **Table 1**) and nearly any substance can be an allergen, with pollens, foods, drugs, and insect venom being common causes of an allergic response. In addition to symptoms directly related to the allergic disease, an immunoglobulin E (IgE)-mediated response to an allergen can exacerbate other chronic conditions, such as asthma and atopic dermatitis. Many patients experience the "atopic march," with the development of atopic dermatitis and food allergies in infancy, followed by asthma, then allergic rhinitis in childhood.[8]

Recently, interest in food allergies has been increasing in the general population.[1] Up to 35% of the general population reports personal belief of a food allergy, although the actual incidence is less than 10%.[1] This erroneous belief can lead to unnecessary avoidance of certain foods. Especially in children this can be problematic, as dietary restrictions can cause problems with weight gain[9] and a decrease in the child's and family's quality of life.[10]

Whereas patients may overdiagnose food allergies, physicians and patients often miss the diagnosis of allergic rhinitis. Often seen as a benign condition, undertreated allergic rhinitis can make asthma control more difficult and have a negative impact on a child's quality of life.[11]

For all types of allergies, therefore, it is important to make an accurate diagnosis using a combination of history, physical examination, and appropriate diagnostic testing. In patients with one atopic disease, physicians may need to probe for symptoms of a second atopic disease (**Box 1**).

Symptom Criteria

IgE-mediated environmental allergies may present with allergic rhinitis or worsening of underlying asthma or atopic dermatitis. Rhinitis is defined as the presence of 1 or more of the following:

- Nasal congestion
- Rhinorrhea (anterior and posterior)
- Sneezing
- Nasal itching[12]

Box 1
Definition of allergies

Allergies are immunologically mediated reactions to a specific allergen (mediated usually, but not always, by immunoglobulin E [IgE]) with symptoms ranging from immediate systemic responses (anaphylaxis) to chronic recurrent symptoms of the respiratory, gastrointestinal, and cutaneous systems.

Individuals are considered allergic when they have both IgE to a specific allergen *and* symptoms that develop after exposure to that substance.

Food allergies are frequently suspected when patients develop either localized symptoms immediately after exposure or systemic symptoms occurring between 5 minutes and 2 hours after exposure.[7] The symptoms are highly variable from patient to patient.

The history is especially important in patients with suspected allergic disease. For example, anaphylaxis 5 minutes after exposure to peanuts on 2 separate occasions is likely to be a true peanut allergy, but hives that develop intermittently, sometimes after eating shellfish, is less likely to be an IgE-mediated allergy. Likewise, for environmental allergies the onset of rhinitis and conjunctivitis during a particular season or after exposure to a furry animal suggests an IgE-mediated allergic component, whereas sneezing after exposure to strong scents suggests a vasomotor or irritant dermatitis.

Food intolerances are often confused with food allergies. Lactose intolerance, which is the genetic absence of the lactase enzyme, is a much more common syndrome than food allergies, and affects up to 70% of the adult population.[13] It is less common in the pediatric population. Gluten intolerance has gained popularity as a potential cause of a variety of symptoms, including gastrointestinal symptoms, fatigue, and migraines.[14] However, the link between gluten intolerance and these symptoms is based on limited data. For both syndromes, testing for IgE-mediated disease will be negative, as there is no allergic component.

CLINICAL FINDINGS
Physical Examination

Physical examination will likely be normal in patients with allergic disease if they have not had a recent exposure. For environmental allergies, examination should focus on the nares, ears, and nasopharynx (**Table 2**).

Rating Scales

Patients with suspected allergic rhinitis should be assessed to determine if symptoms are mild, moderate, or severe, and if they are intermittent or persistent (**Table 3**).[15]

Diagnostic Modalities

The gold standard for diagnosis of food allergies is an observed food challenge (OFC).[16] This test is problematic for several reasons, including unacceptable risk to the patient in cases of anaphylaxis in addition to the expense and time needed to complete the test properly. However, as already stated, it is important to confirm the diagnosis of food allergies rather than to recommend a restrictive diet to pediatric patients.

Therefore, most patients should undergo either a skin-prick test (SPT) or a serum-specific IgE (sIgE) test.[7] Both SPT and sIgE testing will only be positive in patients with an IgE-mediated allergic reaction; patients with other allergic syndromes or intolerances will not have a positive test.[17] Conversely, a positive test for both indicates only the presence of IgE in the system, not a clinical response to the allergen. SPT and sIgE are also appropriate tests in patients with suspected allergic rhinitis.

SPT is a very sensitive test with a high negative predictive value of greater than 90%.[18] Patients are defined as having a positive test if the wheal is larger than 3 mm, and a larger wheal size increases the likelihood that a patient will have an allergic response when exposed to the allergen.[17] However, positive test results can occur in nonallergic patients, and consideration of the patient's history is important when interpreting results. A trained physician must perform the test in a clinical environment, as anaphylaxis is a rare but potential complication.

Table 1
Specific food-induced allergic conditions

Pathology	Disorder	Key Features	Most Common Causal Foods
IgE mediated (acute onset)	Acute urticaria/angioedema	Food commonly causes acute (20%) but rarely chronic urticaria	Primarily major allergens: egg, milk, peanut, fish, soy, wheat
	Contact urticaria	Direct skin contact results in lesions	Multiple
	Anaphylaxis	Rapidly progressive, multiple organ system reaction, can include cardiovascular collapse	Any, more commonly peanut, tree nuts, shellfish, fish, milk, egg
	Food-associated, exercise-induced anaphylaxis	Food triggers anaphylaxis only if ingestion is followed temporally by exercise	Wheat, shellfish, and celery most often described
	Oral allergy syndrome (pollen-associated food allergy syndrome)	Pruritus and mild edema confined to oral cavity; uncommonly progress beyond mouth and rarely to anaphylaxis. Might increase after pollen season	Raw fruit/vegetables; cooked forms tolerated. Examples: birch with apple, pear, peach, carrot, ragweed with melons
	Immediate gastrointestinal hypersensitivity	Immediate vomiting, pain	Major allergens
Combined IgE and cell mediated (delayed onset/ chronic)	Atopic dermatitis	Associated with food allergy in ~35% of children with moderate-to-severe rash	Major allergens, particularly egg, milk
	Eosinophilic esophagitis	Symptoms might include feeding disorders, reflux symptoms, vomiting, dysphagia, and food impaction	Multiple
	Eosinophilic gastroenteritis	Vary on site(s)/degree of eosinophilic inflammation; might include ascites, weight loss, edema, obstruction	Multiple
Cell mediated (delayed onset/ chronic)	Food protein–induced enterocolitis syndrome	Primarily affects infants; chronic exposure: emesis, diarrhea, poor growth, lethargy; reexposure after restriction: emesis, diarrhea, hypotension (1%) 2 h after ingestion	Cow's milk, soy, rice, oat, meat
	Food protein–induced allergic proctocolitis	Mucus-laden, bloody stools in infants	Milk (through breastfeeding)
	Allergic contact dermatitis	Often occupational because of chemical moieties, oleoresins. Systemic contact dermatitis is a rare variant because of ingestion	Spices, fruits, vegetables
	Heinder syndromes	Pulmonary infiltrates, failure to thrive, iron deficiency anemia	Cow's milk

Adapted from Burks AW, Tang M, Sicherer S, et al. ICON: Food allergy. J Allergy Clin Immunol 2012;129(4):908; with permission.

Table 2	
Physical examination in patients with rhinitis	
System	**Specific Evaluation to Perform and Sample Findings**
Vital signs	Weight, height
General	Facial pallor, elongated facies, preferred mouth breathing
Eyes	Excessive lacrimation, erythema and swelling of conjunctiva, swelling or dermatitis of outer eyelids, "allergic shiners"
Nose	Transverse external crease, external deformity, septal deviation or perforation, spurs, ulcers, perforation, prominent vessels, or excoriation; nasal turbinate hypertrophy, edema, pallor or erythema, and crusting; discharge; nasal polyps
Ears	Tympanic membrane dullness, erythema, retraction, perforation, reduced or increased mobility, air-fluid levels
Oropharynx	Halitosis, dental malocclusion, high arched palate, tonsillar or adenoidal hypertrophy, cobblestoning of the oropharyngeal wall, pharyngeal postnasal discharge, temporomandibular joint pain or clicking with occlusion, furrowing, coating, or ulceration of tongue or buccal mucosa
Neck	Lymphadenopathy, thyroid enlargement, or tenderness
Chest	Signs of asthma. Chest wall deformity or tenderness, abnormal percussion, egophony, audible wheezing, or abnormal or diminished sounds by auscultation
Abdomen	Tenderness, distension, masses, or enlargement of liver or spleen
Skin	Rashes, especially eczematous or urticarial, or dermatographism

Adapted from Wallace D, Dykewicz M, Bernstein D, et al. The diagnosis and management of rhinitis: an updated practice parameter. J Allergy Clin Immunol 2008;122(2):S15. http://dx.doi.org/10.1016/j.jaci.2008.06.003; with permission.

Food-specific sIgE levels are more widely available of lower risk to the individual patient. However, sIgE has a lower negative predictive value, as some patients may have a clinical response despite a low positive sIgE.[18] As with SPT and wheal size, higher levels of sIgE are more likely to be associated with a clinically significant allergic reaction. In addition, general panels that test for many allergens may confuse the clinical

Table 3			
Classification of allergic rhinitis			
Intermittent vs Persistent		**Mild vs Moderate/Severe**	
Intermittent	Symptoms present <4 days a week OR for <4 consecutive weeks	Mild	None of the following: • Sleep disturbances • Impairment of daily activities • Impairment of school or work • Symptoms present but not troublesome
Persistent	Symptoms present >4 days a week AND >4 consecutive weeks	Moderate/ Severe	One or more of the following: • Sleep disturbances • Impairment of daily activities • Impairment of school or work • Symptoms present but not troublesome

Adapted from Bousquet J, Khaltaev N, Cruz AA, et al. Allergic Rhinitis and its Impact on Asthma (ARIA) 2008 update (in collaboration with the World Health Organization, GA(2)LEN and AllerGen). Allergy 2008;63:8–160.

picture if patients have a positive test result but a clinical history that is inconsistent with a true allergic disease. The sensitivity, specificity, and reference range of the tests will vary based on the individual laboratory.

Testing for specific allergens should be targeted to the patient's clinical picture. For example, if a patient is known to tolerate eggs, testing for egg allergy will only complicate the diagnosis and may result in unnecessary avoidance. Likewise, environmental allergy testing should focus on the most common allergens (fungi, dust mites, furry animals, and insect emanations) and the types of pollen that are appropriate for the locale and season when patients tend to have symptoms.[12]

Although confirmatory testing should be strongly considered to determine a diagnosis of food allergies, it may not be indicated in patients whose clinical picture strongly suggests allergic rhinitis and respond appropriately to initial clinical treatment. Testing may be appropriate in the following patient scenarios:

- Patients who have a more complicated clinical picture
- Patients who do not respond to treatment
- Patients who are considering immunotherapy

Tests that are not indicated for diagnosis of allergic disease include a total sIgE level, scratch testing, and intradermal skin testing.[7] Atopy patch testing may be appropriate for some patients with environmental allergies, but is not appropriate for diagnosis of food allergies as it has not been standardized (**Table 4**).[15]

MANAGEMENT GOALS

The primary goals of the treatment of both environmental and food allergies are to prevent major complications, such as anaphylaxis and severe asthma exacerbations, and improve overall quality of life. Although pharmacologic treatment will play a role for

Table 4
Diagnostic testing for patients with suspected allergies

Test	Description	Benefits	Risks and Drawbacks
Observed food challenge (OFC)	Patient takes in a small amount of a food that is a suspected allergen in an observed clinical setting	Gold standard for diagnosis	Anaphylaxis Expensive to perform Patient and parent anxiety
Skin-prick testing (SPT)	Skin on forearm is pricked followed by application of droplets of suspected allergens Wheal size is measured	High sensitivity High negative predictive accuracy Immediate results	Low specificity Requires supervision because of low but potential risk for anaphylaxis Requires specialist referral
Serum-specific IgE levels (sIgE)	Enzyme-linked immunosorbent assay test to quantify amount of circulating IgE to a particular antigen	Able to be ordered from physician's office without specialist referral No risk of anaphylaxis	Variable sensitivity and specificity, generally lower than SPT Low false-positive tests may require additional evaluation

Box 2
Treatment of anaphylaxis

In the outpatient setting

First-line treatment:

  Epinephrine IM

    Administer in anterior-lateral thigh

    Epinephrine doses may be repeated every 5 to 15 minutes, as needed

      Autoinjector (EpiPen) dosing:

        Weight 10 to 25 kg: 0.15 mg

        Weight greater than 25 kg: 0.3 mg epinephrine

      Epinephrine, 1:1000 solution

        0.01 mg/kg per dose; maximum dose 0.5 mg per dose

Adjunctive treatment:

  Bronchodilator (β2-agonist) every 20 minutes or continuously as needed

    Albuterol MDI (child: 4–8 puffs; adult: 8 puffs)

    Nebulized solution (child: 1.5 mL; adult: 3 mL)

  H1 antihistamine

    Diphenhydramine (1–2 mg/kg per dose, maximum dose 50 mg IV or oral)

    Oral liquid absorbed more quickly than tablets

    Alternative dosing may be with a less-sedating second-generation antihistamine

  Supplemental oxygen therapy

  IV fluids in large volumes if orthostatic hypotension or incomplete response to IM epinephrine

  Place the patient in recumbent position, if tolerated, with the lower extremities elevated

In the hospital setting

First-line treatment:

  Epinephrine IM

    Administer in anterior-lateral thigh

    Epinephrine doses may be repeated every 5 to 15 minutes, as needed

      Autoinjector (EpiPen) dosing:

        Weight 10 to 25 kg: 0.15 mg

        Weight greater than 25 kg: 0.3 mg epinephrine

      Epinephrine, 1:1000 solution

        0.01 mg/kg per dose; maximum dose 0.5 mg per dose

    Consider continuous epinephrine infusion for persistent hypotension (ideally with continuous noninvasive monitoring of blood pressure and heart rate)

    Alternatives are endotracheal or intraosseous epinephrine

Adjunctive treatment:

  Bronchodilator (β2-agonist) every 20 minutes or continuously, as needed

    Albuterol MDI (child: 4–8 puffs; adult: 8 puffs)

Nebulized solution (child: 1.5 mL; adult: 3 mL)

H1 antihistamine

Diphenhydramine (1–2 mg/kg per dose, maximum dose 50 mg IV or oral)

Oral liquid absorbed more quickly than tablets

Alternative dosing may be with a less-sedating second-generation antihistamine

H2 antihistamine

Ranitidine (1–2 mg/kg per dose, maximum dose 75–150 mg oral and IV)

Corticosteroids

Prednisone at 1 mg/kg with a maximum dose of 60 to 80 mg oral

Methylprednisolone at 1 mg/kg with a maximum dose of 60 to 80 mg

Vasopressors (other than epinephrine) for refractory hypotension

Glucagon for refractory hypotension, titrate to effect

Child: 20 to 30 μg/kg

Adult: 1 to 5 mg

Dose may be repeated or followed by infusion of 5 to 15 μg/min

Atropine for bradycardia, titrate to effect

Supplemental oxygen therapy

IV fluids in large volumes if orthostatic hypotension or incomplete response to IM epinephrine

Place the patient in recumbent position, if tolerated, with the lower extremities elevate

Therapy for the patient at discharge

First-line treatment:

Epinephrine autoinjector prescription (2 doses) and instructions

Education on avoidance of allergen

Follow-up with primary care physician

Consider referral to an allergist

Adjunctive treatment:

H1 antihistamine: diphenhydramine every 6 hours for 2 to 3 days; alternative dosing with a nonsedating second-generation antihistamine

H2 antihistamine: ranitidine twice daily for 2 to 3 days

Corticosteroid: prednisone daily for 2 to 3 days

Abbreviations: IM, intramuscular; MDI, metered-dose inhaler; IV, intravenous.
From Boyce JA, Assa'ad A, Burks AW, et al. Guidelines for the diagnosis and management of food allergy in the United States: summary of the NIAID-Sponsored Expert Panel Report. Nutr Res 2011;31(1):71. http://dx.doi.org/10.1016/j.nutres.2011.01.001; with permission.

many patients, accurate diagnosis and instruction on avoidance techniques are often more important.

Special attention should be paid to the child's overall growth and development when following an avoidance diet. Children with more restrictive diets, especially those with multiple food allergies, may have difficulty with weight gain and the ability to achieve all nutritional requirements.

PHARMACOLOGIC STRATEGIES

There are no current pharmacologic treatments to treat or prevent IgE-mediated allergic reactions to food. Antihistamines, such as diphenhydramine as needed, have a role in the treatment of mild symptoms, such as intermittent urticaria. Allergen-specific immunotherapy for patients with food allergy is an area of investigation,[19] but is not currently recommended for patients with food allergies.[7]

Patients and families should receive instruction on the recognition of anaphylaxis; they should carry an epinephrine autoinjector with them at all times and have adequate instruction on its usage **(Box 2)**.[20]

For patients with allergic rhinitis secondary to environmental allergies there are several treatment options, and consideration should be given to potential side effects, patient's age, and preference. Some are also effective for patients with nonallergic rhinitis, such as irritant arthritis or arthritis resulting from nasal polyps. Other than combinations of oral antihistamines and oral decongestants, there are limited data to support treatment with more than 1 agent.[7] Intranasal corticosteroids are the most effective agents; oral and intranasal antihistamines have a shorter onset of action.[7]

Whereas immunotherapy is not an appropriate treatment for patients with food allergies, it is appropriate for patients with proven environmental allergies for any of the following reasons:

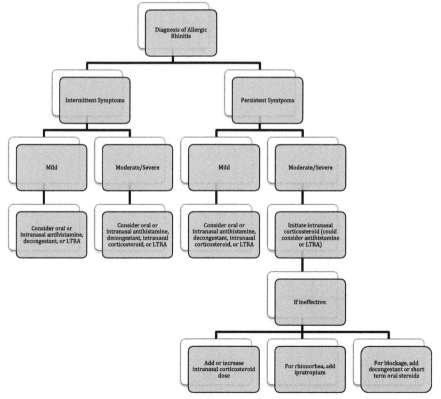

Fig. 1. Treatment algorithm for allergic rhinitis. LTRA, leukotriene receptor antagonist. (*Adapted from* Bousquet J, Khaltaev N, Cruz AA, et al. Allergic Rhinitis and its Impact on Asthma (ARIA) 2008 update (in collaboration with the World Health Organization, GA(2) LEN and AllerGen). Allergy 2008;63:70.)

Table 5
Pharmacologic treatment of allergic rhinitis

Medication	Benefits	Concerning Side Effects	Dosing Per Package Insert	Considerations
Oral Agents				
Oral antihistamines, first generation	Rapid onset of action	Sedation	Diphenhydramine Age 2–5 y: 6.25 mg every 4–6 h as needed; do not exceed 37.5 mg in 24 h Ages 6–11 y: 12.5–25 mg every 4–6 h; do not exceed 150 mg in 24 h Age ≥12 y: 25–50 mg every 4–6 h; do not exceed 300 mg in 24 h	Less effective when primary symptom is nasal congestion
Oral antihistamines, second generation	Rapid onset of action	Fatigue	Fexofenadine Age 6–11 y: 30 mg twice daily Age ≥12 y: 60 mg twice daily or 180 mg daily Loratadine Age 2–5 y: 5 mg daily Age ≥6 y: 10 mg daily Desloratadine Age 2–5 y: 1.25 mg daily Age 6–11: 2.5 mg daily Age ≥12 y: 5 mg daily Cetirizine Age 2–5 y: 2.5–5 mg daily Age ≥6 y: 5–10 mg daily	Ceterizine more sedating than others in class Fexofenadine only available in tablet form
Oral corticosteroids	Effective for very severe nasal symptoms	Weight gain Immunosuppression	Prednisone 1 mg/kg oral; max. dose 60–80 mg	Oral preferable to intramuscular

Oral decongestants	Effective for nasal congestion	Insomnia Irritability Palpitations Hypertension	Pseudoephedrine Age 2–5 y: 15 mg every 4–6 h Age 6–11: 30 mg every 4–6 h Age ≥12 y: 60 mg every 4–6 h	Avoid long-acting pseudoephedrine in children <12 y
Oral leukotriene receptor antagonists	Also approved for treatment of asthma		Montelukast Age 1–2 y: 4 mg daily Age 2–5 y: 4 mg daily Age 6–14 y: 5 mg daily Age ≥12 y: 10 mg daily	May be most appropriate for patients with concomitant asthma and allergic rhinitis Available as granules, tablets, and chewable tablets
Intranasal Agents				
Intranasal antihistamines	Rapid onset of action Better treatment of nasal congestion than oral antihistamines		Azelastine 0.1% Age 5–11 y: 1 spray each nostril daily Age ≥12 y: 2 sprays each nostril daily	Less effective than intranasal corticosteroids Can also treat nonallergic and mixed rhinitis
Intranasal anticholinergics	Rapid onset of action Effective for rhinorrhea	Dry nasal membranes	Ipratropium 0.06% Age 5–11 y: 2 sprays (84 µg) each nostril 3 times daily Age ≥12 y: 2 sprays (84 µg) each nostril 3–4 times daily	
Intranasal corticosteroids	Most effective monotherapy Effective for all symptoms	Nasal irritation Epistaxis Nasal septal	Beclomethasone dipropionate Age ≥6 y: 1–2 sprays each nostril twice daily	Onset of action is slower Can also treat mixed rhinitis

(continued on next page)

Table 5
(continued)

Medication	Benefits	Concerning Side Effects	Dosing Per Package Insert	Considerations
		perforation (rare) Systemic side effects minimal at recommended doses	Budesonide Age 6–11 y: 1–2 sprays each nostril daily Age ≥12 y: 1–4 sprays each nostril daily Ciclesonide Age ≥6 y: 2 sprays each nostril daily Flunisolide Age 6–14 y: 1 spray each nostril 3 times daily or 2 sprays each nostril twice daily Age ≥15 y: 2 sprays each nostril 2–3 times daily Fluticasone furoate Age 2–11 y: 1 spray each nostril daily Age ≥12 y: 2 sprays each nostril daily Fluticasone propionate Age 4–11 y: 1–2 spray each nostril daily Age ≥12 y: 1–2 sprays each nostril daily or 1 spray twice daily Mometasone furoate Age 2–11 y: 1 spray each nostril daily Age ≥12 y: 2 sprays each nostril daily Triamcinolone acetonide Age ≥6 y: 1–2 sprays each nostril daily	
Intranasal cromolyn		Minimal side effects	Cromolyn Age ≥2y: 1 sprays each nostril 3–4 times daily for no more than 12 wk	Can take 4–7 d to see effect; full benefit may take weeks Less effective than intranasal corticosteroids
Intranasal decongestants	May assist in intranasal delivery of other agents if mucosal edema present		Oxymetazoline 0.05% Age ≥6 y: 2–3 sprays each nostril twice daily	Inappropriate for daily use owing to rhinitis medicamentosa

- Inadequate treatment response with other pharmacologic and nonpharmacologic treatments
- Intolerable side effects from other pharmacologic treatments
- Desire to minimize use of daily long-term medications[21]

Allergen immunotherapy, or "allergy shots," involves the injection of a dilution of the allergen 1 to 3 times per week. Patients are started on a lower dilution then gradually titrated up to a maintenance dose over 3 to 6 months, at which point clinical response should be seen (**Fig. 1, Table 5**).[21]

NONPHARMACOLOGIC STRATEGIES

Buffered hypertonic nasal saline irrigation 2 to 3 times daily has been found in several small studies to be effective in reducing allergic symptoms and improving quality of life in pediatric patients with allergic rhinitis.[22,23] It can be administered using a syringe, nasal bulb, or spray, and is generally well tolerated (**Box 3**).[24]

Surgery may be appropriate for patients with severe allergic rhinitis and a comorbid condition such as nasal septal deviation, inferior turbinate hypertrophy, or adenoidal hypertrophy.[12]

SELF-MANAGEMENT STRATEGIES

For both environmental and food allergies, the primary treatment is avoidance. Children with food allergies and their parents may benefit from referral to a nutritionist for assistance in reading food labels and advice on maintaining adequate nutritional intake while avoiding allergens.

Parental education can also help minimize exposure to environmental allergens, which is especially important in controlling symptoms for children who also have asthma.[25,26] Patient education handouts and online resources, such as those listed in **Table 6**, can be especially helpful in guiding patients and their families to minimize exposure to environmental allergens.

Box 3
Buffered hypertonic nasal saline recipe

Mix 3 teaspoons sodium chloride (pickling or canning salt) and 1 teaspoon baking soda.

Add 1 teaspoon of this mixture to 1 cup (8 oz [235 mL]) of lukewarm water that has been boiled or distilled.

EVALUATION, ADJUSTMENT, AND RECURRENCE

As many children with allergies will eventually outgrow their allergies, it is reasonable to consider repeat testing annually or as indicated, based on the patient's individual history. Specifically, most children with food allergies to milk, eggs, soy, and wheat will grow out of their allergies. Children are less likely to outgrow allergies to peanuts, tree nuts, fish, and shellfish.[7] For many children, confirmation that the allergy has resolved may occur after an accidental exposure. The decision to pursue an observed oral challenge should be made based on the wheal size for patients undergoing SPT or sIgE levels, and should likely be made in concert with an allergist.[7]

Table 6
Patient education handouts for environmental and food allergies

Source	Website
Family Doctor (from American Family Physician)	http://familydoctor.org/familydoctor/en/diseases-conditions/allergic-rhinitis.html http://familydoctor.org/familydoctor/en/diseases-conditions/food-allergies.html
National Allergy Bureau (NAB) Pollen Counts	http://www.aaaai.org/global/nab-pollen-counts.aspx
American Academy of Allergy, Asthma, and Immunology (AAAAI)	http://www.aaaai.org/conditions-and-treatments/library/at-a-glance/indoor-allergens.aspx http://www.aaaai.org/conditions-and-treatments/allergies/food-allergies.aspx
Food Allergy Research and Education (FARE)	http://www.foodallergy.org/
Consortium on Food Allergy Research (CoFAR)	http://cofargroup.org/

For allergic rhinitis, treatment outcomes should be reassessed after 2 to 4 weeks,[15] at which point it may be reasonable to consider the following:

- An increase in dose, or
- Addition of a second agent if there is inadequate symptom relief, or
- Discontinuation of therapy in patients with intermittent allergic rhinitis who have had a resolution of symptoms

SUMMARY

Allergic disease is common. For food allergies the incidence is increasing, although the exact prevalence is difficult to ascertain, as self-reported allergies are more common than clinically confirmed food allergies. On the other hand, allergic rhinitis is often unrecognized and undertreated. Primary care physicians play an important role in disease recognition, patient education, monitoring the growth and development of patients with allergic disease, and initial management of allergic rhinitis, with specialty consultation as appropriate for disease confirmation and management.

REFERENCES

1. Rona RJ, Keil T, Summers C, et al. The prevalence of food allergy: a meta-analysis. J Allergy Clin Immunol 2007;120(3):638–46. http://dx.doi.org/10.1016/j.jaci.2007.05.026.
2. Blackwell DL, Tonthat L. Summary health statistics for US Children: National Health Interview Survey, 1999. Vital Health Stat 10 2003;(210):1–50. Available at: http://eric.ed.gov/?id=ED478700. Accessed February 18, 2014.
3. Gupta RS, Springston EE, Warrier MR, et al. The prevalence, severity, and distribution of childhood food allergy in the United States. Pediatrics 2011;128(1):e9–17. http://dx.doi.org/10.1542/peds.2011-0204.
4. Björkstén B, Clayton T, Ellwood P, et al, ISAAC Phase III Study Group. Worldwide time trends for symptoms of rhinitis and conjunctivitis: Phase III of the International Study of Asthma and Allergies in Childhood. Pediatr Allergy Immunol 2008;19(2):110–24. http://dx.doi.org/10.1111/j.1399-3038.2007.00601.x.

5. Sicherer SH, Muñoz-Furlong A, Godbold JH, et al. US prevalence of self-reported peanut, tree nut, and sesame allergy: 11-year follow-up. J Allergy Clin Immunol 2010;125(6):1322–6. http://dx.doi.org/10.1016/j.jaci.2010.03.029.

6. Osborne NJ, Koplin JJ, Martin PE, et al. Prevalence of challenge-proven IgE-mediated food allergy using population-based sampling and predetermined challenge criteria in infants. J Allergy Clin Immunol 2011;127(3):668–76.e1-2. http://dx.doi.org/10.1016/j.jaci.2011.01.039.

7. Boyce JA, Assa'ad A, Burks AW, et al. Guidelines for the diagnosis and management of food allergy in the United States: summary of the NIAID-sponsored expert panel report. Nutr Res 2011;31(1):61–75. http://dx.doi.org/10.1016/j.nutres.2011.01.001.

8. Spergel J. Atopic dermatitis and the atopic march. J Allergy Clin Immunol 2003; 112(6):S118–27. http://dx.doi.org/10.1016/j.jaci.2003.09.033.

9. Flammarion S, Santos C, Guimber D, et al. Diet and nutritional status of children with food allergies: nutritional status of food allergic children. Pediatr Allergy Immunol 2011;22(2):161–5. http://dx.doi.org/10.1111/j.1399-3038.2010.01028.x.

10. Cummings AJ, Knibb RC, King RM, et al. The psychosocial impact of food allergy and food hypersensitivity in children, adolescents and their families: a review: the psychosocial impact of food allergy. Allergy 2010;65(8):933–45. http://dx.doi.org/10.1111/j.1398-9995.2010.02342.x.

11. Stewart MG. Identification and management of undiagnosed and undertreated allergic rhinitis in adults and children. Clin Exp Allergy 2008;38(5):751–60. http://dx.doi.org/10.1111/j.1365-2222.2008.02937.x.

12. Wallace D, Dykewicz M, Bernstein D, et al. The diagnosis and management of rhinitis: an updated practice parameter. J Allergy Clin Immunol 2008;122(2): S1–84. http://dx.doi.org/10.1016/j.jaci.2008.06.003.

13. Lomer MC, Parkes GC, Sanderson JD. Review article: lactose intolerance in clinical practice - myths and realities. Aliment Pharmacol Ther 2007;27(2):93–103. http://dx.doi.org/10.1111/j.1365-2036.2007.03557.x.

14. Biesiekierski JR, Muir JG, Gibson PR. Is gluten a cause of gastrointestinal symptoms in people without celiac disease? Curr Allergy Asthma Rep 2013;13(6): 631–8. http://dx.doi.org/10.1007/s11882-013-0386-4.

15. Bousquet J, Khaltaev N, Cruz AA, et al. Allergic Rhinitis and its Impact on Asthma (ARIA) 2008 update (in collaboration with the World Health Organization, GA(2) LEN and AllerGen). Allergy 2008;63:8–160. http://dx.doi.org/10.1111/j.1398-9995.2007.01620.x.

16. Du Toit G, Santos A, Roberts G, et al. The diagnosis of IgE-mediated food allergy in childhood. Pediatr Allergy Immunol 2009;20(4):309–19. http://dx.doi.org/10.1111/j.1399-3038.2009.00887.x.

17. Lieberman JA, Sicherer SH. Diagnosis of food allergy: epicutaneous skin tests, in vitro tests, and oral food challenge. Curr Allergy Asthma Rep 2010;11(1): 58–64. http://dx.doi.org/10.1007/s11882-010-0149-4.

18. Sicherer SH, Sampson HA. Food allergy. J Allergy Clin Immunol 2010;125(2): S116–25. http://dx.doi.org/10.1016/j.jaci.2009.08.028.

19. Sabato V, Faber M, Van Gasse A, et al. State of the art and perspectives in food allergy (part II): therapy. Curr Pharm Des 2014;20(6):964–72.

20. Sicherer SH, Sampson HA. Food allergy: epidemiology, pathogenesis, diagnosis, and treatment. J Allergy Clin Immunol 2014;133(2):291–307.e5. http://dx.doi.org/10.1016/j.jaci.2013.11.020.

21. Cox L, Nelson H, Lockey R, et al. Allergen immunotherapy: a practice parameter third update. J Allergy Clin Immunol 2011;127(1):S1–55. http://dx.doi.org/10.1016/j.jaci.2010.09.034.

22. Khianey R, Oppenheimer J. Is nasal saline irrigation all it is cracked up to be? Ann Allergy Asthma Immunol 2012;109(1):20–8. http://dx.doi.org/10.1016/j.anai. 2012.04.019.

23. Satdhabudha A, Poachanukoon O. Efficacy of buffered hypertonic saline nasal irrigation in children with symptomatic allergic rhinitis: a randomized double-blind study. Int J Pediatr Otorhinolaryngol 2012;76(4):583–8. http://dx.doi.org/ 10.1016/j.ijporl.2012.01.022.

24. AAAAI. Saline sinus rinse allergy treatment recipe. Available at: https://www. aaaai.org/conditions-and-treatments/library/allergy-library/saline-sinus-rinse-recipe.aspx. Accessed March 13, 2014.

25. Crain EF, Walter M, O'Connor GT, et al. Home and allergic characteristics of children with asthma in seven US urban communities and design of an environmental intervention: the Inner-City Asthma Study. Environ Health Perspect 2002;110(9):939.

26. Morgan WJ, Crain EF, Gruchalla RS, et al. Results of a home-based environmental intervention among urban children with asthma. N Engl J Med 2004; 351(11):1068–80.

Pediatric Asthma for the Primary Care Practitioner

Anne VanGarsse, MD[a],*, Richard D. Magie, DO, RPh[a], Aubree Bruhnding, BS[b]

KEYWORDS

- Asthma • Pediatrics • Primary care practitioner • Guidelines

KEY POINTS

- Asthma is a common chronic inflammatory disease of the airways.
- It is a complex disease, involving many different allergic, inflammatory, and environmental components.
- It is a disease for which patient and family education and a team-based approach are paramount for successful management.
- National Guidelines have been put forth by the National Heart, Lung and Blood Institute, which provide a helpful framework to begin to manage patients and to navigate the many medication choices available.
- It is only through diligent attention to control of asthma symptoms that improved quality of life and prevention of long-term sequelae are possible for the pediatric patient with asthma.

INTRODUCTION

In the mid to late twentieth century, asthma was defined as a disease characterized by an increased responsiveness of the trachea and bronchi to various stimuli and manifested by widespread airway narrowing that changed in severity either spontaneously or as a result of treatment. This definition is no longer complete enough to define asthma in the twenty-first century.

Asthma affects at least 24 million individuals in the United States and is the most common chronic inflammatory disease of childhood (at least 7 million children are affected). In the pediatric world of medicine, males have a higher prevalence of asthma. African Americans and Puerto Ricans have the highest prevalence compared with whites and Mexican-Americans. Those who compose lower socioeconomic status are at increased risk, as are those in the Northeast United States.[1]

The authors have nothing to disclose.
[a] Department of Pediatrics, College of Osteopathic Medicine, Kansas City University of Medicine, 1750 Independence Avenue, Kansas City, MO 64106, USA; [b] College of Osteopathic Medicine, Kansas City University of Medicine and Biosciences, 1750 Independence Avenue, Kansas City, MO 64106, USA
* Corresponding author.
E-mail address: avangarsse@kcumb.edu

Prim Care Clin Office Pract 42 (2015) 129–142
http://dx.doi.org/10.1016/j.pop.2014.09.013
0095-4543/15/$ – see front matter © 2015 Elsevier Inc. All rights reserved.

By definition, asthma is the result of inflammation of the airways and narrowing of the airways, which is at least in part reversible. It occurs in paroxysms, causing symptoms of cough, wheezing, chest tightness, and difficulty breathing. Episodes are related to increased responsiveness of the airways to a variety of stimuli. Once believed to be entirely caused by bronchospasm of the smooth muscles lining the airways, asthma is viewed as a more complex chronic disease.

Medical information has greatly increased as science and biomedical research have enabled a more complete understanding of the disease processes of asthma. The incidence of disease has continued to increase, but the rate of acute attacks of asthma has remained constant over the past few years. According to the US Centers for Disease Control and Prevention 2006 National Health Interview Survey, there is a lifetime asthma prevalence of 13.5%.[2]

The components of asthma resulting in the symptoms and clinical expression of asthma include inflammation, edema (swelling), airway narrowing (secondary to edema, muscle thickening, and muscle contraction), airway plugging (secretions, inflammatory cells/debris), and basement membrane thickening caused by type IV collagen deposition.

The purpose of this article is to improve understanding of the basics and methods of the treatment of children with asthma.

PATHOPHYSIOLOGY OF ASTHMA

Asthma is a chronic inflammatory disease of the airways, characterized by varying and recurrent symptoms of airway obstruction, hyperresponsiveness, and underlying inflammation.[3] Asthma manifests clinically as intermittent and recurrent wheezing or coughing.

In children, there are 2 main categories of asthma:

1. Recurrent wheezing (also called intrinsic asthma)
   - This typically arises from nonallergic causes
   - In early childhood, asthma is mostly caused by viral respiratory infections[3]
   - Can also be caused by aspirin/nonsteroidal antiinflammatory drug sensitivity
   - Some patients are also sensitive to environmental irritants, such as air pollutants, smoke, stress, exercise, and cold air
2. Chronic asthma (also called allergic or extrinsic asthma)
   - Mediated by a type 1 hypersensitivity reaction

Although there are distinct types of asthma, airway inflammation, hyperresponsiveness, and excess production of mucus are ubiquitous and are the result of a complex inflammatory response.

INFLAMMATORY RESPONSE
Inflammatory Cells and Their Roles

Lymphocytes, specifically T helper 1 (Th1) and T helper 2 (Th2), have distinct regulatory mechanisms that affect airway function.[4]
- A shift toward Th2 cells results in eosinophil recruitment and inflammation.
- Th2 release cytokines such as interleukin 4 (IL-4) and IL-5.
- Regulatory T cells, which normally inhibit Th2 cells and stimulate natural killer cells, are reduced, contributing to the lack of regulatory control over the Th2 response.
- Mast cells in the mucosa become activated from cross-linking of the increased IgE levels, and release histamine, leukotrienes C4/D4/E4 and prostaglandin D_2.

- These inflammatory mediators cause bronchoconstriction, mucous production, and edema.

Generally, an increase in eosinophils correlates to increasing asthma severity.

Neutrophils are increased in the airways and sputum of severe asthmatics during exacerbations.

- Their pathologic role is uncertain, but neutrophils may explain a lack of response to corticosteroid therapy.
- They are the predominant cell type present in the airways of patients with nonallergic (intrinsic) asthma.[5]

Dendritic cells function as antigen-presenting cells, presenting the allergens from the airway to the regional lymph nodes.

- In the lymph nodes, these cells interact with regulatory T cells, resulting in the stimulation of Th2 cells from naive T cells.

Macrophages are present in the highest amounts in asthmatic airways and are activated by allergens to release inflammatory cytokines.

Airway smooth muscle cells also contribute to airway obstruction through generating their own proinflammatory cells.

- When the smooth muscle proliferates and hypertrophies, this response is accelerated, contributing to the disease process.

These inflammatory cellular infiltrates and exudates also obstruct the airways. They are capable of causing damage to the epithelium and even desquamation into the airway lumen.[4]

Inflammatory Mediators and Their Roles

IgE is the antibody responsible for starting a type I hypersensitivity reaction.

- IgE attaches to high-affinity receptors on the cell surfaces.
- Mast cells express IgE receptors in large amounts, as well as basophils, dendritic cells, and lymphocytes.
- Clinical findings in the development of monoclonal antibodies to IgE support the understood role of IgE in asthma.

Chemokines (eotaxin) are expressed in airway cells and work to recruit inflammatory cells.

Cytokines control the inflammatory response in asthma and directly influence its severity.

- Th2 releases cytokines IL-4 and IL-5, which leads to eosinophil recruitment and the overproduction of IgE.
- Other Th2 cytokines include IL-1 and tumor necrosis factor α, which amplify the inflammatory response, and granulocyte macrophage colony-stimulating factors, which promote eosinophil survival.

Leukotrienes C4/D4/E4 released by mast cells along with histamine and prostaglandin D_2 are potent bronchoconstrictors.

These inflammatory cells and mediators result in hyperresponsiveness, leading to bronchospasm and constriction of the airways, as well as mucous production and airway edema.

As mentioned earlier, it is hypothesized that an imbalance between Th1 and Th2 cells, resulting in a shift toward Th2 cytokine profiles, contributes to the disease process. There may be a loss of the reciprocal relationship between Th1 and Th2, an underexpression of Th1, or overexpression of Th2.[6]

Several factors favor the development of a protective Th1 phenotype, such as the presence of older siblings, early exposure to day care, a rural environment, and infections such as tuberculosis, measles, or hepatitis A. Alternatively, a Western lifestyle, urban environment, house-dust mite sensitization, widespread antibiotic use, and diet can contribute to a Th2 phenotype, which can result in allergic diseases and asthma.

Respiratory infections during infancy have been associated with the development of asthma, as well. Respiratory syncytial virus (RSV) and parainfluenza virus cause bronchiolitis, which manifests similarly to childhood asthma.[3]

Although some studies show that such infections confer a risk (approximately 40%) of wheezing or asthma later in life,[4] evidence also shows that repeated viral infections, including RSV, can help develop a strong Th1 response and protect against asthma. Research is focused on understanding the innate and adaptive immune process and interplay with genes and environment.

EPIDEMIOLOGY

Asthma is a common chronic disease, causing considerable morbidity. Current prevalence in the United States has been reported to be 8.2% up to 2010.[1] This prevalence includes 24.6 million people, 7.1 million of whom are children from birth to 17 years of age.

This statistic represents an overall increase in the prevalence of asthma since 2001, when current measures first began. In 2001, prevalence was 7.4% and remained fairly stable until recent increases to current prevalence of 8.2%.[1] Although the incidence of asthma has stabilized, the prevalence still remains at an all-time high.

Prevalence of asthma differs between multiple subgroups of the population.

- Prevalence of current asthma for children is higher overall, at 9.6%, than for adults, at 7.7%.
- Children ages 14 to 17 years have similar prevalence for both genders.
- Gender difference becomes reversed from childhood (11.3% of boys vs 7.9% of girls).
- During early adolescence, asthma prevalence declines steadily in boys and increases steadily for girls.
- Adult women have a higher prevalence of asthma overall, with 9.3% of women having asthma, compared with 7% of men.
- Current asthma prevalence is also higher for African Americans, Puerto Ricans, and those with family incomes lower than the federal poverty level.
- Prevalence for metropolitan and nonmetropolitan areas does not differ.
- Regional differences in prevalence are also noted, with higher rates in the Northeast and Midwest regions of the United States.[1]
- Prevalence of asthma attacks among people with asthma is 52%, as of 2009,[7] defined as patients having had at least 1 attack in the previous year.[7]
- Fifty-six percent of children with asthma reported attacks.[7]
- Forty-seven percent of adults with asthma reported attacks.[7]

Data from a 2008 aggregate report[1] show that children aged 5 to 17 years who suffered at least 1 asthma attack in the previous year were reported to have missed a total of 10.5 million days of school in that year. In addition, 5.5% of children with asthma reported activity limitations caused by their asthma.

Adults with asthma during the same period who also reported at least 1 attack in the previous year missed a total of 14.2 million work days, with 34% missing at least 1 day of work because of their asthma and 6% experiencing an activity limitation.[1]

Health care use and costs for asthma are high. In 2007, 13.9 million visits were made to physician offices for asthma, with 6.7 million of those visits including treatment of children with asthma.[1] This situation may represent some measure of appropriate disease management, because periodic health maintenance visits for management are recommended. However, emergency department (ED) visits and hospital admissions for asthma represent adverse outcomes, and 1.75 million ED visits for asthma were reported during the same period; 640,000 of these were for children aged 0 to 17 years, and 157,000 hospital admissions were reported for children that year, with 185 deaths.[1]

In 2008, 96% of patients with a current asthma diagnosis reported that a health care team member provided education about proper inhaler use, but only 34% reported receiving a written asthma action plan with instructions about (1) increasing medication dosage, (2) changing medicines, or (3) when to call a medical provider and when to proceed to the ED for emergent care.

Sixty percent reported receiving education on recognizing personal signs and symptoms of an asthma attack. When compared with adults, children reported a higher rate of receiving asthma control instructions.[6]

Just as the cause of asthma is not understood, the complex role of asthma self-management, including environmental exposures, health care system access, and financial factors, is not well understood. Identifying any population-specific factors that contribute to asthma attacks or prevent their timely treatment can lead to targeted interventions for that population.[7]

TREATMENT
Four Components of Asthma Care

The clinical practice guidelines for diagnosis and management of asthma, as put forth by the National Heart Lung and Blood Institute Expert Panel Report 4, published in 2007, present 4 components for effective asthma care.[6]

Component 1: measures of asthma assessment and monitoring
Component 2: education and partnership in asthma care
Component 3: control of environmental factors and comorbid conditions affecting asthma
Component 4: pharmacologic management

Component 1: assessing and monitoring asthma severity, control, and responsiveness
Step 1: making the diagnosis
Diagnosing the pediatric patient is the first step toward eliminating the symptoms and improving quality of life and preventing long-term sequelae.
- A detailed medical history and physical examination, with a focus on the upper respiratory tract, chest, and skin
- Spirometry use in conjunction helps diagnose asthma and rule out other diagnoses

Clinical features suggestive of asthma diagnosis[4]:
- History of episodic or chronic airway obstruction symptoms that are at least partially reversible
- Response to and duration of albuterol
- Spirometry before administration of bronchodilator:
    FEV_1 (forced expiratory volume in first second of expiration) less than 80% predicted, FEV_1/forced vital capacity less than 85%
- Spirometry after administration of bronchodilator:
    $FEV \geq 9\%$ from baseline, showing reversible airway obstruction
- Exclusion of alternative diagnoses

Ancillary studies may include a methacholine challenge in patients with symptoms suggestive of asthma but normal spirometry, chest radiograph to rule out congenital malformations, sweat chloride test to rule out cystic fibrosis, barium swallow for patients with reflux, and allergy testing for environmental allergens in very young children.

In children younger than 5 years, the diagnostic process remains the same; however, spirometry may be unavailable. Asthma is a chronic condition, whereas nonatopic conditions like wheezy bronchitis and virus-induced wheezing tend to resolve by the age of 5 years.

Step 2: assessing the severity Although severity is most easily measured in a patient not on long-term treatment, if a patient is already receiving medication, the severity can be inferred from the amount of treatment needed to maintain control.

Figs. 1 and **2**, from the Expert Panel,[1] show how to classify asthma severity in pediatric patients, based on age groups.

In patients not on long-term controller medications and for children of all ages, experiencing symptoms 2 days a week, or if the patient's classification changes

Classifying severity in children who are not currently taking long-term control medication.

Components of Severity		Classification of Asthma Severity (Children 0–4 years of age)			
			Persistent		
		Intermittent	Mild	Moderate	Severe
Impairment	Symptoms	≤2 days/week	>2 days/week but not daily	Daily	Throughout the day
	Nighttime awakenings	0	1–2x/month	3–4x/month	>1x/week
	Short-acting beta₂-agonist use for symptom control (not prevention of EIB)	≤2 days/week	>2 days/week but not daily	Daily	Several times per day
	Interference with normal activity	None	Minor limitation	Some limitation	Extremely limited
Risk	Exacerbations requiring oral systemic corticosteroids	0–1/year	≥2 exacerbations in 6 months requiring oral steroids, or ≥4 wheezing episodes/1 year lasting >1 day AND risk factors for persistent asthma		
		Consider severity and interval since last exacerbation. Frequency and severity may fluctuate over time.			
		Exacerbations of any severity may occur in patients in any severity category			

Fig. 1. Classification of asthma severity in children aged 0 to 4 years. EIB, exercise-induced bronchospasm. Level of severity is determined by both impairment and risk. Assess impairment domain by caregiver's recall of previous 2–4 weeks. Assign severity to the most severe category in which any feature occurs. At present, there are inadequate data to correspond frequencies of exacerbations with different levels of asthma severity. For treatment purposes, patients who had ≥2 exacerbations requiring oral corticosteroids in the past 6 months, or ≥4 wheezing episodes in the past year, and who have risk factors for persistent asthma may be considered the same as patients who have persistent asthma, even in the absence of impairment levels consistent with persistent asthma. (*From* National Asthma Education and Prevention Program. Expert Panel report 3 (EPR3): guidelines for the diagnosis and management of asthma. Bethesda (MD): National Heart, Lung and Blood Institute; 2007. (NIH publication no 08-4051). Available at: http://www.nhlbi.nih.gov/guidelines/asthma/asthgdln.htm.)

Classifying severity in children who are not currently taking long-term control medication.

Components of Severity		Classification of Asthma Severity (Children 5–11 years of age)			
		Intermittent	Persistent		
			Mild	Moderate	Severe
Impairment	Symptoms	≤2 days/week	>2 days/week but not daily	Daily	Throughout the day
	Nighttime awakenings	≤2x/month	3–4x/month	>1x/week but not nightly	Often 7x/week
	Short-acting beta$_2$-agonist use for symptom control (not prevention of EIB)	≤2 days/week	>2 days/week but not daily	Daily	Several times per day
	Interference with normal activity	None	Minor limitation	Some limitation	Extremely limited
	Lung function	• Normal FEV$_1$ between exacerbations • FEV$_1$ >80% predicted • FEV$_1$/FVC >85%	• FEV$_1$ = >80% predicted • FEV$_1$/FVC >80%	• FEV$_1$ = 60–80% predicted • FEV$_1$/FVC = 75–80%	• FEV$_1$ <60% predicted • FEV$_1$/FVC <75%
Risk	Exacerbations requiring oral systemic corticosteroids	0–1/year (see note)	≥2 in 1 year (see note) → ← Consider severity and interval since last exacerbation. Frequency and severity may fluctuate over time for patients in any severity category. → Relative annual risk of exacerbations may be related to FEV$_1$		

Fig. 2. Classification of asthma severity in children aged 5 to 11 years. EIB, exercise-induced bronchospasm; FEV$_1$, forced expiratory volume in second; FVC, forced vital capacity; ICU, intensive care unit. Level of severity is determined by both impairment and risk. Assess impairment domain by patient's/caregiver's recall of the previous 2–4 weeks and spirometry. Assign severity to the most severe category in which any feature occurs. At present, there are inadequate data to correspond frequencies of exacerbations with different levels of asthma severity. In general, more frequent and intense exacerbations (e.g., requiring urgent, unscheduled care, hospitalization, or ICU admission) indicate greater underlying disease severity. For treatment purposes, patients who had ≥2 exacerbations requiring oral systemic corticosteroids in the past year may be considered the same as patients who have persistent asthma, even in the absence of impairment levels consistent with persistent asthma. (*From* National Asthma Education and Prevention Program. Expert Panel report 3 (EPR3): guidelines for the diagnosis and management of asthma. Bethesda (MD): National Heart, Lung and Blood Institute; 2007. (NIH publication no 08-4051). Available at: http://www.nhlbi.nih.gov/guidelines/asthma/asthgdln.htm.)

from intermittent to persistent, then, the frequency of symptoms greater than 2 days a week determines the patient's classification within the persistent categories.

For pediatric patients already on controller treatment, the lowest level of treatment that is needed to keep them in control determines their classification status.

Although initial diagnosis is crucial, after diagnosis, the focus of care must shift to long-term control and therapeutic responsiveness.

The goals are the same for every patient with asthma, despite varying baseline severity, and are as follows:

Periodic assessment is recommended every 1 to 6 months to assess if therapeutic goals are being met and to make modifications if needed.

Clinicians should encourage the patient or patient's family to keep a daily diary or fill out a periodic self-assessment form as a way of self-monitoring.

In children younger than 4 years, the clinician is encouraged, by the Expert Panel, to refer the patient to a specialist in asthma care, if after 3 to 6 months, the patient does not meet asthma therapy goals or requires step 3 or higher in children (**Figs. 3** and **4**) younger than 4 years.

Major goals of asthma therapy
1. Reduce impairment
   - Prevent chronic and recurrent symptoms, such as coughing or breathlessness
   - Require infrequent use (<2 days a week) of inhaled short-acting β-agonist
   - Maintain near normal pulmonary function
   - Maintain normal activity levels, including exercise and school attendance
   - Meet patients' and families' expectations of asthma care
2. Reduce risk
   - Prevent recurrent exacerbations and minimize need for ED visits and hospitalizations
   - Prevent reduced lung growth in children
   - Provide optimal pharmacologic therapy with minimal or no adverse effects

Component 2: education for partnership in asthma care

Education in self-management of asthma is crucial to provide patients and their families with the necessary skills to achieve asthma control and improve long-term outcomes.

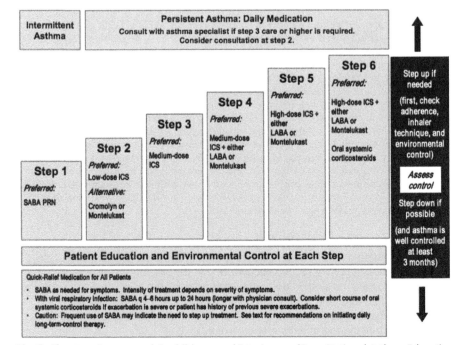

Fig. 3. The stepwise approach in children aged 0 to 4 years. (*From* National Asthma Education and Prevention Program. Expert Panel report 3 (EPR3): guidelines for the diagnosis and management of asthma. Bethesda (MD): National Heart, Lung and Blood Institute; 2007. (NIH publication no 08-4051). Available at: http://www.nhlbi.nih.gov/guidelines/asthma/asthgdln.htm.)

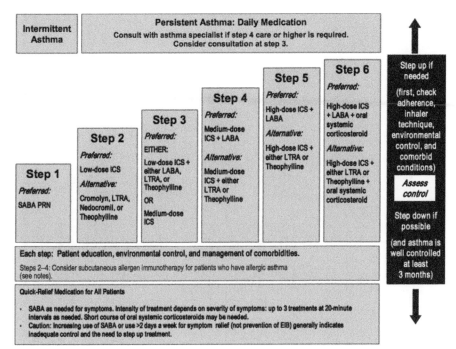

Fig. 4. The stepwise approach in children aged 5 to 11 years. ICS, inhaled corticosteroids; LABA, long-acting β-agonists; PRN, as needed; SABA, short-acting β-agonists. (*From* National Asthma Education and Prevention Program. Expert Panel report 3 (EPR3): guidelines for the diagnosis and management of asthma. Bethesda (MD): National Heart, Lung and Blood Institute; 2007. (NIH publication no 08-4051). Available at: http://www.nhlbi.nih.gov/guidelines/asthma/asthgdln.htm.)

- This education should begin when a diagnosis of asthma is first made and continue at each subsequent visit.
- To facilitate this goal, the Expert Panel[6] recommends that clinicians provide all patients with a written asthma action plan (**Fig. 5**).
- The plan should include daily management strategies and tips for recognizing exacerbations.

Key components of the written asthma action plan should include:

- Which medicines to take daily, including their specific names
- Ways to control environmental factors that exacerbate the patient's asthma
- Explicit ways to recognize and handle worsening symptoms and the medications to take in response
- Conditions for which the patient should seek emergent medical care, and the telephone numbers for the physician and ED

Component 3: control of environmental factors and comorbid conditions that affect asthma

There is a strong relationship between asthma and allergy, especially indoor allergens. Patients experience increased asthma exacerbations and symptoms when exposed to allergens to which they are sensitive.[6]

In addition, studies show that sensitization to indoor allergens, such as animal dander, house-dust mite, and cockroaches, is an established risk for developing

Asthma Action Plan

For: _____   Doctor: _____   Date: _____

Doctor's Phone Number _____   Hospital/Emergency Department Phone Number _____

Doing Well

GREEN ZONE

- No cough, wheeze, chest tightness, or shortness of breath during the day or night
- Can do usual activities

And, if a peak flow meter is used,

Peak flow: more than _____
(80 percent or more of my best peak flow)

My best peak flow is: _____

Take these long-term control medicines each day (include an anti-inflammatory).

Medicine	How much to take	When to take it
Before exercise	⊓ 2 or ⊓ 4 puffs	5 minutes before exercise

Asthma Is Getting Worse

YELLOW ZONE

- Cough, wheeze, chest tightness, or shortness of breath, or
- Waking at night due to asthma, or
- Can do some, but not all, usual activities

-Or-

Peak flow: _____ to _____
(50 to 79 percent of my best peak flow)

First Add: quick-relief medicine—and keep taking your GREEN ZONE medicine.

_____ (short-acting beta₂-agonist)   ⊓ 2 or ⊓ 4 puffs, every 20 minutes for up to 1 hour
                                        ⊓ Nebulizer, once

Second **If your symptoms (and peak flow, if used) return to GREEN ZONE after 1 hour of above treatment:**
- ⊓ Continue monitoring to be sure you stay in the green zone

-Or-

If your symptoms (and peak flow, if used) do not return to GREEN ZONE after 1 hour of above treatment:
- ⊓ Take: _____ (short-acting beta₂-agonist)   ⊓ 2 or ⊓ 4 puffs or ⊓ Nebulizer
- ⊓ Add: _____ (oral steroid)   _____ mg per day For _____ (3–10) days
- ⊓ Call the doctor ⊓ before/ ⊓ within _____ hours after taking the oral steroid.

Medical Alert!

RED ZONE

- Very short of breath, or
- Quick-relief medicines have not helped, or
- Cannot do usual activities, or
- Symptoms are same or get worse after 24 hours in Yellow Zone

-Or-

Peak flow: less than _____
(50 percent of my best peak flow)

Take this medicine:

⊓ _____ (short-acting beta₂-agonist)   ⊓ 4 or ⊓ 6 puffs or ⊓ Nebulizer
⊓ _____ (oral steroid)   _____ mg

Then call your doctor NOW. Go to the hospital or call an ambulance if:
- You are still in the red zone after 15 minutes AND
- You have not reached your doctor.

DANGER SIGNS ■ **Trouble walking and talking due to shortness of breath**   ■ **Take ⊓ 4 or ⊓ 6 puffs of your quick-relief medicine AND**
              ■ **Lips or fingernails are blue**   ■ **Go to the hospital or call for an ambulance** _____ **NOW!**
                                                                                                              (phone)

Fig. 5. The written asthma action plan. (*From* National Asthma Education and Prevention Program. Expert Panel report 3 (EPR3): guidelines for the diagnosis and management of asthma. Bethesda (MD): National Heart, Lung and Blood Institute; 2007. (NIH publication no 08-4051). Available at: http://www.nhlbi.nih.gov/health/public/lung/asthma/asthma_actplan.pdf.)

asthma as a child. Outdoor pollen sensitization is less of a risk; however, ragweed and grass can be associated with seasonal asthma. It is crucial to eliminate, or significantly reduce, exposure to inhaled allergens.[6]

- The clinician can evaluate the role of allergens through obtaining a medical history of allergen exposure and skin testing or in vitro testing to determine sensitivity in the context of patient history.
- The first and most important step in controlling allergen-induced asthma is to reduce exposure in a multifaceted approach.
- A multistep process that includes all environments is most effective. Single steps are typically not effective. Precautions should be taken in the home, as well as other environments, like school or daycare.
- Families can contact the Asthma and Allergy Foundation of America toll-free hotline at 800-727-8462 or the Allergy and Asthma Network/Mothers of Asthmatics at 800-878-4403 for information about companies with products to help reduce allergen exposure.

All patients with asthma should avoid:

- Exposure to allergens to which the patient has documented sensitivities
- Exposure to environmental tobacco smoke and smoke from wood-burning stoves and fireplaces
- Outdoor exertion when air pollution levels are high
- Use of nonselective β-blockers
- Sulfite-containing foods and other foods to which they are sensitized
- Use of humidifiers and evaporative coolers in patient's home if there are known sensitivities to house-dust mites or mold
- Occupational exposures
- Dealing with household pets can be a difficult topics to address. If the patient is sensitive to the animal, the treatment of choice is to remove the animal from the home. However, if this is not an option, patients should keep the pet out of the bedroom and keep the door closed. Upholstered furniture and carpets should be removed, or pet access to those areas of the home should be limited.
- House-dust mites can be controlled by encasing the mattress and pillow in an impermeable cover or by weekly pillow washing. Sheets and blankets should be washed weekly in hot water, at a temperature greater than 130°F. Cockroach allergen can be reduced if patients and their families do not leave food and garbage exposed and focus on intensive cleaning of the home.
- Immunotherapy can be considered in patients showing clear evidence of symptoms after exposure to an antigen. Immunotherapy should be administered only in a physician's office, with trained personnel and available equipment to treat any life-threatening event, which, although rare, can occur.

Component 4: pharmacologic management

Asthma medications are categorized into long-term control medications used to achieve and maintain control of persistent asthma and quick-relief medications for acute symptoms and asthma exacerbations. Both categories of medications are listed in alphabetical order in **Tables 1** and **2**.

The most comprehensive approach to managing asthma in patients of all ages is the stepwise approach, outlined in the Expert Panel.[6] The stepwise approach has been tailored for patients ages 0 to 4 years, 5 to 11 years, and those 12 years or older. The approach is intended to supplement but not replace the clinician's judgment and can be tailored to meet the patient's needs.

Table 1
Long-term medications

Long-Term Medications	Mechanism	Indications
Corticosteroids	Block late-phase reaction to allergens, reduce airway hyperresponsiveness, and inhibit inflammatory cell activation	Inhaled corticosteroids (ICS) are the most potent and effective antiinflammatory medications available, used in severe persistent asthma
Cromolyn sodium and nedocromil	Stabilizes mast cells and interferes with chloride channel function	Alternative treatment of mild persistent asthma or prophylactic treatment of exercise
Immunomodulators	Omalizumab (anti-IgE) is a monoclonal antibody that prohibits IgE from binding to receptors on basophils and mast cells	Adjunctive therapy for patients $\geq$12 y old with allergies and severe persistent asthma, monitor patients after injection for anaphylaxis
Leukotriene modifiers	Montelukast (patients >1 y) and zafirlukast (patients >7 y) are leukotriene receptor antagonists, zileuton is 5-lipoxygenase pathway inhibitor (patients $\geq$12 y)	Alternative treatment option for mild persistent asthma, or as alternative adjunct to ICS when a LABA is not appropriate Monitor liver function in zileuton
LABA	Salmeterol and formoterol bronchodilate for $\geq$12 h	Used in combination with ICS for long-term control in moderate or severe persistent asthma in children $\geq$5 y
Methylxanthines	Sustained-released theophylline, mild to moderate bronchodilator	Alternative, not preferred, adjunctive therapy with ICS Monitor serum concentration

Abbreviations: ICS, inhaled corticosteroids, LABA, long-acting β-agonists.

- Pharmacologic management of childhood asthma is challenging, because children rarely stay in a single classification from season to season. This situation means that parental and patient education about their medications is an essential component.

Table 2
Quick-relief medications

Quick-Relief Medications	Mechanism	Indications
Anticholinergics	Inhibit muscarinic cholinergic receptors and reduce vagal tone	Alternative bronchodilator for patients who cannot tolerate a SABA
SABA	Albuterol, levalbuterol, and pirbuterol bronchodilate and relax smooth muscle	Therapy of choice for acute symptom relief and prevention of exercise-induced bronchospasm
Systemic corticosteroids		Moderate and severe exacerbations, as adjunct to SABA to speed recovery

Abbreviation: SABA, short-acting β-agonits.

- In addition, patient and parent education about use of devices can be a challenge, because children perceive being different (ie, needing medication) as not being socially accepted by their peers.
- Once a patient has been classified into a category, decisions concerning their directed therapy must be made in conjunction with parental and patient input. Therapy works only if there is buy-in by the patient or parent.
- First, consider a child who has intermittent asthma. This patient is best treated with a quick-acting inhaled β_2-selective adrenergic agonist, taken at the time that symptoms appear. The goal is to treat the intermittent symptoms, not prevent them.
- In addition, patient education concerning recognition of triggers of the symptoms is important to aid in avoidance of the use of medication.
- The medication of choice for most of the patients in this category or classification is albuterol sulfate via inhalation (other choices are levalbuterol, or if the child is $\geq$12 years of age, pirbuterol).
- In the United States, there are rarely indications for the use of oral quick-acting bronchodilators.
- Patient education is important to ensure that the medication is being delivered to the affected airways. In children, especially those younger than 4 years, a spacer with a mask is the most appropriate delivery method. Spacers should be encouraged for children of all ages if available.
- Close follow-up is necessary to monitor the patient's symptoms, assess for the need to adjust therapy, search for environmental triggers, and to continue patient education, especially over the first few months of therapy.
- If a child with apparent intermittent asthma has the need for systemic corticosteroids twice or more in a 6-month period, the child should be treated as a child with a persistent form of asthma.
- In young children (especially those <12 months old), the use of a home nebulizer may be considered. Many families with older children who have abrupt exacerbations of their asthma are more comfortable with having a nebulizer as an additional or alternative means of providing rescue medication to their children.
- The child who is classified as having persistent asthma is at more risk for having symptoms that wax and wane, from the mild or moderate categories to the severe category during certain seasons.
- The initial additional medication for children in a category of persistent asthma is the addition of a controller medication. Much has been reported about the benefits of controller medications, especially inhaled corticosteroids.
- In the age of information and Internet availability, many patients' parents have some information and an opinion of the use of the benefits and risks of inhaled corticosteroids.

The use of a low-dose inhaled corticosteroid is recommended for initial therapy in children with apparent mild persistent asthma (budesonide is the only product approved for children <4 years of age).

If there is parental resistance to the use of steroids as controller medication, especially in the mild persistent category, an alternative is the use of a leukotriene receptor antagonist (LTRA) (montelukast has been approved for use to treat rhinitis in children aged $\geq$6 months and is the most commonly used LTRA in children in the United States).

So, in children younger than 4 years, the use of budesonide is recommended, with the alternative being the use of montelukast in children older than 1 year (in whom it has been approved for use to control asthma symptoms). If inhaled corticosteroids are used, we suggest rinsing of the oral cavity (or brushing of teeth) after each use.

The asthmatic child classified in the moderate persistent category should be treated with a medium daily dose of inhaled corticosteroids. Again, therapy should be closely monitored initially to assess control of symptoms. For children not controlled on medium doses of inhaled corticosteroids, an evaluation by an asthma specialist (pulmonologist or allergist) should be strongly considered by the primary care physician.

SUMMARY

Asthma is a common chronic inflammatory disease of the airways. It affects at least 7 million children in the United States, with more than 150,000 annual pediatric hospital admissions and 185 pediatric deaths.[1] It is a complex disease, involving many different allergic, inflammatory, and environmental components. Patient and family education and a team-based approach are paramount for successful management of the disease. National guidelines have been put forth by the National Heart, Lung and Blood Institute, which provide a helpful framework in which to begin to manage patients and to navigate the many medication choices available. It is only through diligent attention to control of asthma symptoms that improved quality of life and prevention of long-term sequelae are possible for the pediatric asthma patient.

REFERENCES

1. Akinbami L, Moorman J, Liu X. Asthma prevalence, health care use and mortality: United States, 2005-2009. National Health Statistics Reports. US Department of Health and Human Services; Hyattsville (MD): Centers for Disease Control and Prevention; 2011 (32).
2. Bloom B, Cohen RA, Freeman G. Summary health statistics for U.S. children: National Health Interview Survey, 2007. Vital Health Stat 10 2009;(239):1–80. Available at: http://www.cdc.gov/nchs.htm. Accessed November 22, 2013.
3. Liu AH, Covar RA, Spahn JD, et al. Childhood asthma. In: Kliegman RM, editor. Nelson textbook of pediatrics. 19th edition. Philadelphia: Elsevier; 2011. p. 780–5.
4. Robinson DS. The role of the T cell in asthma. J Allergy Clin Immunol 2010;126: 1081.
5. Simpson J, Scott R, Boyle M, et al. Inflammatory subtypes in asthma: assessment and identification using induced sputum. Respirology 2006;11:54–61.
6. National Asthma Education and Prevention Program. Expert Panel report 3 (EPR3): guidelines for the diagnosis and management of asthma. Bethesda (MD): National Heart, Lung and Blood Institute; 2007 (NIH publication no 08-4051). Available at: http://www.nhlbi.nih.gov/guidelines/asthma/asthgdln.htm.
7. Moorman JE, Person CJ, Zahran HS, Centers for Disease Control and Prevention (CDC). Asthma attacks among persons with current asthma–United States 2001-2010. MMWR Surveill Summ 2013;62(Suppl 3):93–8.

Pediatric Hypertension
A Growing Problem

Debra Ahern, DO[a],*, Emily Dixon, DO[b]

KEYWORDS

- Pediatric hypertension • Pediatric obesity • Pediatric screening • Pediatric workup
- Pediatric lifestyle change

KEY POINTS

- Hypertension in children and adolescents, once thought to be rare, has been estimated at a current prevalence of between 1% and 5% in the United States.
- The frequency of hypertension in children can be expected to increase along with the occurrence of metabolic syndrome as childhood obesity rates rise.
- Many issues are still controversial, but the issue cannot be ignored.
- While systematic reviews and guidelines are in process, clinicians must follow the best evidence available to monitor and treat this related disorder.

INTRODUCTION: A GROWING PROBLEM

Hypertension in children and adolescents, once thought to be rare, has been estimated at a current prevalence of between 1% and 5% in the United States. Most estimates are derived from school screening studies among junior or high school students.[1] Among children younger than 6 years, 83% had secondary hypertension, with renal or renovascular disease the most common comorbidity.[1] In this age category, the children were less likely to be obese and more likely to have elevations in their diastolic pressures. Primary hypertension is more likely to be diagnosed in older children and adolescents. The prevalence of primary hypertension continues to increase with the increasing body mass index (BMI) of the pediatric population, a phenomenon documented in Asia, Europe, and Latin America as well as in the United States.[2] It is estimated that the prevalence of hypertension among obese children in the United States is 11%.[3]

In contrast to the adult population, in which absolute values of diastolic and systolic readings define the diagnosis of hypertension, blood pressure measurements in

The authors have nothing to disclose.
[a] Department of Community and Family Medicine, TMC Lakewood, 7900 Lee's Summit Road, Kansas City, MO 64139, USA; [b] Bethesda Family Practice and Sports Medicine Fellowship, Tri-health Orthopedic and Spine Institute, 8311 Montgomery Rd, Cincinnati, OH 45236, USA
* Corresponding author.
E-mail address: debra.ahern@tmcmed.org

children steadily increase as the child grows, varies with gender, and must be interpreted by referring to data collected from 70,000 healthy children in the United States. The measurements in this national database are organized into percentiles based on age, gender, and height.[4] A child is considered normotensive if both the systolic and diastolic readings are below the 90th percentile, and is considered prehypertensive if the systolic or diastolic pressures reach the 90th percentile but are less than the 95th percentile or reach 120/80 mm Hg. Stage 1 pediatric hypertension is diagnosed when the measurements are at or above the 95th percentile but less than the 99th percentile plus 5 mm Hg. Values exceeding the 99th percentile plus 5 mm Hg define stage 2 pediatric hypertension.[5]

Recommendations for blood pressure screening in asymptomatic children are controversial. The American Heart Association National Heart, Lung and Blood Institute[6] expert panel recommends annual screening blood pressures for children between the ages of 3 and 17 years.[3] The American Academy of Pediatrics recommends screening of children ages 3 years and older at every "health care episode." By contrast, the United States Preventive Services Task Force and the American Academy of Family Practice state that there is insufficient evidence for or against routine screening for high blood pressure in this age group.[3]

THE FIRST QUESTION THAT MUST BE ANSWERED: IS THE PATIENT TRULY HYPERTENSIVE?

The gathering of accurate data is an essential part of any diagnosis, and several pitfalls must be avoided when monitoring blood pressures in the pediatric population.

First, the proper cuff size must be selected. The cuff bladder width should span at least 40% of the upper extremity circumference measured halfway between the elbow and the shoulder, while its length should cover 80% to 100% of the circumference. If a cuff is too small it will overestimate blood pressure readings. If 2 sizes of cuff appear to meet these criteria, the larger cuff should be used.

Systolic or diastolic readings that exceed the 90th percentile by automatic (oscillometric) devices should be confirmed by auscultation after the patient has been seated for 5 minutes with the back supported and the feet uncrossed on the floor. Pressures should be evaluated in the right arm supported at the level of the heart. Two readings should be done and averaged together. In one study of 390 children, 74% had significantly lower blood pressures when data were gathered by trained personnel using the Fourth Task Force recommendations than those obtained using an automated device at the vital signs station.[7]

During the initial screening, it is important to assess for coarctation of the aorta. Blood pressures should be measured in both arms while the child is seated and in one leg with the patient prone. Pressures should be 10 to 22 mm Hg higher in the leg but approximately equal in the arms. Femoral pulses should also be assessed. Coarctation of the aorta should be suspected when pressures in the left arm are significantly lower than in the right upper extremity, the expected higher pressure is not found in the leg, or the femoral pulses are diminished.[8]

Patients whose blood pressure remains elevated should be brought back for further evaluation. The diagnosis of prehypertension or hypertension is confirmed when the readings remain elevated on 3 separate occasions at least 1 week apart. A study of 1071 9- to 10-year-olds in Iceland found the prevalence of elevated blood pressures to be 13.1% at the first screen, 6% at the second screen, and 3.1% at the third screen.[2] In a study of more than 6000 adolescents in Hong Kong, the prevalence of elevated blood pressures similarly decreased from 9.54% at the first evaluation to 1.44% by the third assessment.[2]

Ambulatory blood pressure monitoring (ABPM) should be considered in the setting of intermittent elevated blood pressures, when the diagnosis of white-coat hypertension is being considered or when the caregiver reports normal blood pressures outside of the clinic. ABPM typically involves 2 to 4 blood pressures per hour over a 24-hour period. Mean diurnal and nocturnal blood pressures are then calculated. Children who fail to exhibit the expected 10% decline in readings during sleep should be further evaluated for renal scarring. ABPM may also be used to assess the effectiveness of treatment.[9]

PEDIATRIC HYPERTENSION: WHO IS AT RISK?

The genetic basis of pediatric hypertension is poorly understood but is likely to be polygenetic in most cases. However, single gene defects have increasingly been identified in this population. Male gender and African American ethnicity both increase the propensity toward elevated pressures.[3,8]

The dramatic increase in both prehypertension and hypertension in children, as in adults, has been linked directly to the increase rate of obesity.[3,10] Insulin resistance and sleep abnormalities have been independently shown to contribute to hypertension. It has been hypothesized that adiposity might accelerate the development of hypertension in children with genetic predispositions.[10]

In 2011 Raj[10] reviewed several studies that confirmed the relationship between uric acid levels higher than 5.5 mg/dL and elevated blood pressures in adolescents.[3,10] A recent placebo-controlled study by Soletsky and Feig demonstrated that adolescents with elevated uric acid levels who were treated with allopurinol or probenecid for 2 months had a significant lowering of their blood pressure.[11] Further studies must be done before treatment of uric acid levels as a treatment for elevated blood pressures can be recommended.

Breast feeding has been shown in multiple studies to have a small, but statistically significant, protective effect in patients who were breastfed as infants, having lower systolic and diastolic pressures later in childhood.[12]

Smoking or exposure to secondhand smoke and increased time spent in sedentary activities have been independently linked with elevated pressures in children, as has lower socioeconomic status.[13]

Prematurity and low birth weights have been identified as risk factors for the development of pediatric hypertension.[10] It has been hypothesized that this may be due to smaller kidney size and fewer numbers of nephrons. A history of umbilical catheterization, which increases the risk for renal artery stenosis, has also been linked to the development of hypertension in children.[10] A history of maternal preeclampsia or eclampsia are further risk factors.[13]

LONG-TERM IMPLICATIONS OF PEDIATRIC HYPERTENSION: SO WHAT ARE WE WORRIED ABOUT?

Although there is no direct evidence that screening asymptomatic children for hypertension will prevent cardiovascular disease in adulthood, there is evidence that elevated blood pressures, starting at age 5, track into adulthood.[13] Almost half of adults with hypertension were found to have elevated blood pressures as children.

Evidence of target organ damage from elevated pressures is also concerning. Echocardiography confirms that almost half of adolescents with hypertension have left ventricular mass indices (LVMIs) above the 90th percentile, and 14% have LVMIs that exceed the 99th percentile.[13] Left ventricular hypertrophy is more common in obese hypertensive youths than in patients with similar BMIs that were normotensive. Increased pressures in children have also been linked to increases in carotid intima-media thickness, which is hypothesized to be a marker of early cardiovascular disorder.[13]

Evidence of hypertensive retinopathy has been documented in patients as young as 6 years of age.

Microalbuminuria, a sign of early renal damage, has also been found in pediatric hypertensive patients. It is especially common in obese black adolescents with hypertension.

Several studies have found impaired cognitive function in pediatric patients with elevated blood pressures. Learning disabilities and attention problems have also been documented, with some evidence of improvement with treatment of the blood pressures.[13]

THE WORKUP: DIFFERENTIATING BETWEEN PRIMARY AND SECONDARY HYPERTENSION

Overweight adolescents who present with prehypertension or stage 1 hypertension are most likely to be diagnosed with primary hypertension, whereas secondary hypertension is most frequently found in the young child or the patient with stage 2 hypertension. Because renovascular or renal parenchymal abnormality is found in 10% of pediatric hypertensive patients, it is important to thoroughly evaluate all children with elevated pressures. Although the Fourth Task Force recommended that young children undergo more extensive evaluation for renovascular disease, they failed to specify an age cutoff for this workup. Various studies have found increased probabilities of secondary causes of hypertension in children younger than 12 years, 10 years, and 6 years.[14] Nonobese younger patients with elevated diastolic pressures and lower glomerular filtration rates are most likely to be diagnosed with renovascular disorder.

As in every good evaluation, a complete history should be obtained with emphasis on birth history (gestational age, birth weight, history of umbilical artery catheterization). Patients or caregivers should be queried about a history of urinary tract infections, sleep difficulties, and symptoms of end-organ damage such as palpitations, chest pain, dizziness, headaches, and so forth. A medication history should be obtained that includes the use of herbal products, energy drinks, and illegal substances.

A careful physical examination should be performed with emphasis on auscultation of the heart and the abdomen (seeking evidence of abdominal bruits). If not previously done, blood pressures should be taken in both arms and one leg to evaluate for coarctation of the aorta. A fundoscopic examination to rule out retinal abnormalities is also important.

Initial laboratory tests should include electrolytes, blood urea nitrogen, and creatinine, and a urine dipstick seeking evidence of proteinuria. Urine dipsticks become positive when urine albumin exceeds 330 mg/d. There is no current recommendation that routine assessment for microalbuminemia need be done in the asymptomatic pediatric patient with hypertension.[14]

An ultrasonogram of the kidneys should be obtained to look for small kidney sizes and unilateral kidneys. Renal scarring may or may not be evident on ultrasonography. Doppler evaluation of the renal vessels should be limited only to those patients in whom there is a high suspicion of renal abnormality, including patients with Williams syndrome, Marfan syndrome, neurofibromatosis, or tubular sclerosis, and those whose blood pressures are not adequately controlled on multiple medications.

Owing to the high rates of left ventricular hypertrophy in this population, an echocardiogram should be obtained. Echocardiograms are also useful to confirm the diagnosis of coarctation of the aorta.

Adolescents with normal lab tests, ultrasonogram, and echocardiogram on the initial evaluation should be diagnosed with primary hypertension.

Further evaluations for less prevalent causes of pediatric hypertension, such as hyperthyroid disease and pheochromocytoma, should be performed only if clinically indicated.

TREATMENT OF PEDIATRIC HYPERTENSION

The treatment of pediatric hypertension should be aimed at the cause. However, with the obesity epidemic and the increase in the number of pediatric and adolescent patients diagnosed with metabolic syndrome, preventing hypertension in these populations is paramount. For both primary and secondary hypertension, exacerbating factors, such as poor dietary and physical activity habits, smoking, stress, sleep disturbance, and obesity, should be addressed and minimized.[7]

The Fourth Report Task Force outlines an algorithm for the management of hypertension (**Fig. 1**). The goal is to reduce blood pressure to within the normal range while preventing or reversing target end-organ damage.[4] Patients with secondary hypertension usually require management by specialists in the underlying etiology. A pediatric patient who requires pharmacologic management will often benefit from consultation with a pediatric hypertension specialist, often a cardiologist or nephrologist.

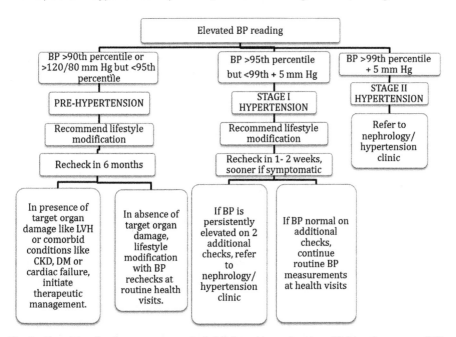

Fig. 1. Algorithm for the management of childhood hypertension. BP, blood pressure; CKD, chronic kidney disease; DM, diabetes mellitus; LVH, left ventricular hypertrophy. (*From* Anyaegbu EI, Dharnidharka VR. Hypertension in the teenager. Pediatr Clin North Am 2014;61(1):138; with permission.)

Behavioral and lifestyle changes are the initial treatment option for management of hypertension and prehypertension. Weight reduction and weight management are key components in this process. Specific health behaviors include targeted dietary modifications, increased levels of physical activity, decreased time in sedentary pursuits, and the elimination of exposure to tobacco smoke.[15] A meta-analysis of clinical trials in children and adolescents by Kelley and colleagues[16] found a 1% reduction in systolic blood pressure and 3% reduction in diastolic blood pressure with exercise interventions, although these findings were not statistically significant.

The American Academy of Pediatrics (AAP) recommends a goal of at least 60 minutes of moderate to strenuous physical activity daily. The AAP also recommends a reduction of sedentary activities, including restricting screen time to less than 2 hours per day.[17] Often adolescents are found to have elevated blood pressures at their annual preparticipation sports evaluation. For primary hypertension the treatment is often exercise. However, athletes who have severe hypertension, characterized as greater than 5 mm Hg over the 99th percentile for age, sex, and height, should be disqualified from sports that require a high static demand, and should also avoid heavy weight training and powerlifting.[15] Patients with uncontrolled stage 2 hypertension should be restricted from participation in all competitive sports.

Dietary modifications aimed at obesity and the overweight individuals should include a reduction of cholesterol and fat intake in addition to a reduction of sweetened drinks and processed fast foods. Increasing the intake of fresh fruits and vegetables, limiting portion size and snacking, and eating meals as a family are all to be encouraged. Saneei and colleagues[18] found that a modified Dietary Approach to Stop Hypertension (DASH) diet for 6 weeks in adolescents reduced the prevalence of high blood pressure. The macronutrient composition of the modified DASH diet was as follows: carbohydrates, 53% to 58%; proteins, 15% to 8%; total fats, 26% to 30% of total energy. The DASH diet contained less than 2400 mg Na/d and contained high amounts of whole grains, fruits, vegetables, and low-fat dairy products, and low amounts of saturated fats, cholesterol, refined grains, sweets, and red meat.[18]

Pharmacologic management is reserved for patients who fail behavioral modification, or who have stage 1 or 2 hypertension. The presence of other comorbidities such as hyperlipidemia or diabetes, which increase cardiovascular risk, should be a further indication for pharmacologic treatment. The goal is to reduce blood pressure to below the 95th percentile and to prevent target organ damage.[7] Several classes of drugs have been used to treat pediatric and adolescent patients with hypertension. However, there are no studies that compare different drugs in children and, as a result, guidelines about the use of specific agents are vague.

Several classes of drugs are suitable for management, including angiotensin-converting enzyme (ACE) inhibitors, angiotensin-receptor blockers (ARB), β-blockers, calcium-channel blockers, and diuretics. Flynn and Daniels[19] reviewed the pediatric dosing information for these medications. The choice of initial drug is at the discretion of the provider. For patients with comorbidities such as diabetes or proteinuric renal disease, an ACE inhibitor or ARB may be appropriate. Calcium-channel blockers or β-blockers are often used as prophylaxis for migraines, so they may be preferred in these cases. Non-cardioselective β-blockers should be avoided in patients with asthma, as they may trigger an attack or counteract the effect of a β2-agonist used to counter an asthma attack. The key to pharmacologic management is to start at the lowest dose possible and titrate up to response. A stepwise, individualized approach is recommended. Hypertensive emergencies are rare in children and are often related to other comorbidities. Hypertensive emergencies should be managed in the inpatient setting, with intravenous medications administered by a specialist.[20]

SUMMARY

The frequency of hypertension in children can be expected to increase along with the occurrence of metabolic syndrome as childhood obesity rates rise. Many issues are still controversial, but the issue cannot be ignored. While systematic reviews and guidelines are in process, clinicians must follow the best evidence available to monitor and treat this related disorder.

ACKNOWLEDGMENTS

The authors would like to thank Gwen E. Sprague, MLS, the Clinical Medical Librarian at Truman Medical Center Lakewood Medical-Dental Library, for her assistance in the literature review and editing process for this article.

REFERENCES

1. Lande MB, Kupferman JC. Pediatric hypertension: the year in review. Clin Pediatr (Phila) 2014;53(4):315–9. http://dx.doi.org/10.1177/0009922813499968.
2. Malatesta-Muncher R, Mitsnefes MM. Management of blood pressure in children. Curr Opin Nephrol Hypertens 2012;21(3):318–22. http://dx.doi.org/10.1097/MNH. 0b013e328351c415.
3. Moyer VA, U.S. Preventive Services Task Force. Screening for primary hypertension in children and adolescents: U.S. Preventive Services Task Force recommendation statement. Ann Intern Med 2013;159(9):613–9. http://dx.doi.org/10. 7326/0003-4819-159-9-201311050-00725.
4. National High Blood Pressure Education Program Working Group on High Blood Pressure in Children and Adolescents. The fourth report on the diagnosis, evaluation, and treatment of high blood pressure in children and adolescents. Pediatrics 2004;114(2 Suppl 4th Report):555–76.
5. Stephens MM, Fox BA, Maxwell L. Therapeutic options for the treatment of hypertension in children and adolescents. Clin Med Insights Circ Respir Pulm Med 2012;6:13–25. http://dx.doi.org/10.4137/CCRPM.S7602.
6. Chapter 8, Pediatric cardiovascular risk reduction guidelines, NHLBI. Available at: http://www.nhlbi.nih.gov/guidelines/cvd_ped/chapter8.htm. Accessed May 6, 2014.
7. McCrindle BW. Assessment and management of hypertension in children and adolescents. Nat Rev Cardiol 2010;7(3):155–63. http://dx.doi.org/10.1038/nrcardio. 2009.231.
8. Anyaegbu EI, Dharnidharka VR. Hypertension in the teenager. Pediatr Clin North Am 2014;61(1):131–51. http://dx.doi.org/10.1016/j.pcl.2013.09.011.
9. Sanders JT, Jones DP. Work up of the child with hypertension. J Med Liban 2010; 58(3):156–60.
10. Raj M. Essential hypertension in adolescents and children: recent advances in causative mechanisms. Indian J Endocrinol Metab 2011;15(Suppl 4):S367–73. http://dx.doi.org/10.4103/2230-8210.86981.
11. Soletsky B, Feig DI. Uric acid reduction rectifies prehypertension in obese adolescents. Hypertension 2012;60(5):1148–56.

12. Martin RM, Gunnell D, Smith GD. Breastfeeding in infancy and blood pressure in later life: systematic review and meta-analysis. Am J Epidemiol 2005;161(1): 15–26. http://dx.doi.org/10.1093/aje/kwh338.

13. Bucher BS, Ferrarini A, Weber N, et al. Primary hypertension in childhood. Curr Hypertens Rep 2013;15(5):444–52. http://dx.doi.org/10.1007/s11906-013-0378-8.

14. Kapur G, Baracco R. Evaluation of hypertension in children. Curr Hypertens Rep 2013;15(5):433–43. http://dx.doi.org/10.1007/s11906-013-0371-2.

15. Peterson AR, Bernhardt DT. The preparticipation sports evaluation. Pediatr Rev 2011;32(5):e53–65. http://dx.doi.org/10.1542/pir.32-5-e53.

16. Kelley GA, Kelley KS, Tran ZV. The effects of exercise on resting blood pressure in children and adolescents: a meta-analysis of randomized controlled trials. Prev Cardiol 2003;6(1):8–16.

17. Council on Sports Medicine and Fitness, Council on School Health. Active healthy living: prevention of childhood obesity through increased physical activity. Pediatrics 2006;117(5):1834–42. http://dx.doi.org/10.1542/peds.2006-0472.

18. Saneei P, Hashemipour M, Kelishadi R, et al. Effects of recommendations to follow the dietary approaches to stop hypertension (DASH) diet v. usual dietary advice on childhood metabolic syndrome: a randomised cross-over clinical trial. Br J Nutr 2013;110(12):2250–9. http://dx.doi.org/10.1017/S0007114513001724.

19. Flynn JT, Daniels SR. Pharmacologic treatment of hypertension in children and adolescents. J Pediatr 2006;149(6):746–54. http://dx.doi.org/10.1016/j.jpeds. 2006.08.074.

20. Patel HP, Mitsnefes M. Advances in the pathogenesis and management of hypertensive crisis. Curr Opin Pediatr 2005;17(2):210–4.

Addressing Obesity with Pediatric Patients and Their Families in a Primary Care Office

Carlene A. Mayfield, MPH[a],*, Richard R. Suminski, PhD, MPH[b]

KEYWORDS

- Pediatric obesity • Treatment • Diet • Exercise

KEY POINTS

- Overweight is defined as a BMI at or above the 85th percentile and lower than the 95th percentile for children of the same age and sex; obesity is defined as a BMI that is at or above the 95th percentile for children of the same age and sex.
- Children and teenagers that are overweight or obese should focus on weight maintenance or weight loss, depending on several key factors.
- The US Department of Agriculture/US Department of Health and Human Services recommend a diet rich in fruits and vegetables, whole grains, and fat-free and low-fat dairy products for persons aged 2 years and older.
- Children should be advised to perform 60 or more minutes of physical activity each day.
- Behavior therapy can be an important adjunct treatment of weight loss and weight maintenance.

INTRODUCTION

Obesity is a major health problem in the United States. Since first recognized as a chronic disease by the National Institutes of Health in 1985, childhood obesity has more than doubled in children and quadrupled in adolescents in the past 30 years.[1] According to the National Center for Health Statistics, the percentage of US children in the 6 to 11 age group who were obese increased from 7% in 1980 to nearly 18% in 2012. Similarly, the percentage of adolescents in the 12 to 19 age group who were obese has increased from 5% to 21% over the same time period.[2] Furthermore, overweight and obese children are more likely to become and stay obese into adulthood[3] and more likely to develop noncommunicable diseases, such as diabetes and

[a] Department of Physiology, 454 SEP, Kansas City University of Medicine and Biosciences, 1750 Independence Ave., Kansas City, MO 64109, USA; [b] Department of Physiology, 454 SEP, Kansas City University of Medicine and Biosciences, Kansas City, MO 64109, USA
* Corresponding author.
E-mail address: cmayfield@kcumb.edu

Prim Care Clin Office Pract 42 (2015) 151–157
http://dx.doi.org/10.1016/j.pop.2014.09.008
0095-4543/15/$ – see front matter © 2015 Elsevier Inc. All rights reserved.

cardiovascular disease, at a younger age.[4] With the prevalence of childhood obesity and overweight in today's society, the family physician must be comfortable counseling parents of obese and overweight children about treatment options. This article discusses the diagnosis and treatment of obesity with an emphasis on diet, physical activity, pharmacotherapy, gastric bypass, and behavior therapy.

DIAGNOSING OBESITY AND OVERWEIGHT

Body mass index (BMI; weight [kg]/height squared [m^2], or weight [lb]/height squared [in] * 703) can be used to assess a person's weight as it relates to their height. For children weight status is further conceptualized as a BMI percentile, which is determined by plotting BMI on a normal curve according a child's age and gender. The Centers for Disease Control and Prevention has developed growth charts that define overweight as a BMI at or above the 85th percentile and lower than the 95th percentile for children of the same age and sex.[5] Obesity is defined as a BMI that is at or above the 95th percentile for children of the same age and sex.[5]

TREATMENT: GENERAL GUIDELINES

After determining that a patient is obese and organic causes are ruled out, a treatment plan should be established. First, the physician must determine if contraindications to weight loss programs exist. When considering weight-reduction programs, patients often have unrealistic expectations, hoping to achieve weight loss goals within a short period of time.[6] This can be a source of disappointment and frustration. The National Institutes of Health/National Heart, Lung, and Blood Institute recommend that children and teenagers that are overweight or obese should focus on weight maintenance or weight loss, depending on several factors.[7] Healthy youth are expected to gain weight as they grow taller, so an obese child that maintains their current weight will still reflect positive health changes in some circumstances. **Table 1** describes the different factors to consider when determining a patient's treatment goals.[8] It is important for physicians to educate parents about this and align patient expectations with what is known to be realistic to avoid the patient having feelings of failure and parent frustration.

The main strategies for weight loss and weight maintenance are dietary therapy; physical activity; combined therapy; pharmacotherapy; and weight loss surgery,

Table 1
Factors to consider when determining treatment outcome goals

Goal: Weight Maintenance	Goal: Weight Loss
All children at risk for becoming overweight (BMI >85th percentile and <95th percentile) between 2 and 7 y of age with no medical complications	All obese children (BMI ≥95th percentile) older than 7 y
Obese children (BMI ≥95th percentile) between 2 and 7 y of age with no medical complications	Obese children between 2 and 7 y with medical complications
	Children at risk for becoming overweight (BMI >85th percentile and <95th percentile) older than 7 y with medical complications

Adapted from Fowler-Brown A, Kahwati LC. Prevention and treatment of overweight in children and adolescents. Am Fam Physician 2004;69(11):2597.

also known as bariatric surgery.[9] Treatment modalities are most successful when approached in a combined fashion.[10] For example, diet and physical activity together achieve a greater success rate than diet alone.

DIETARY THERAPY

The US Department of Agriculture/US Department of Health and Human Services recommend a diet rich in fruits and vegetables, whole grains, and fat-free and low-fat dairy products for persons aged 2 years and older. The guidelines also recommend that children and adolescents limit intake of solid fats (major sources of saturated and trans fatty acids), cholesterol, sodium, added sugars, and refined grains.[11] **Table 2** provides the US Department of Agriculture/US Department of Health and Human Services caloric recommendations for children and adolescents based on age, gender, and activity level. It should be noted that the caloric data are presented in a range where the lower end could support weight loss and the higher end could support weight maintenance depending on the individual needs of the patient.

Patients should determine their caloric intake by filling out a daily food diary, and then adjust their total intake as described. Web sites and mobile phone applications have been created to assist in completing the food diary. Most women lose weight with 1000 to 1200 kcal/d and men with 1200 to 1600 kcal/d. Calories can be increased by 100 to 200 kcal/d if the patient is hungry. Very-low-calorie diets are not recommended because they require close monitoring and nutrient supplementation. It is recommended that more than half of the calories (55%) come from complex carbohydrates, 15% from protein, and less than 30% from fat. Cholesterol, sodium, calcium, and fiber should also be monitored. Cholesterol intake should be less than 300 mg/d; sodium, less than 2.4 g/d; calcium, 1000 to 1500 mg/d; and fiber, 20 to 30 g/d.

PHYSICAL ACTIVITY

Increasing physical activity is critical for obesity prevention, long-term weight maintenance, and overall improvements in health.[12,13] The US Preventive Services Task Force recommends that all patients seen in a primary care setting be advised to reduce dietary fat consumption and increase physical activity.[14] Although physicians can substantially impact patient activity levels,[15] many physicians do not have the time for exercise counseling during the average patient visit.[16] This problem can be

Table 2
Estimated calorie needs per day by age, gender, and physical activity level

| Gender | Age (y) | Physical Activity Level | | |
		Sedentary	Moderately Active	Active
Child (male or female)	2–3	1000–1200	1000–1400	1000–1400
Female	4–8	1200–1400	1400–1600	1400–1800
	9–13	1400–1600	1600–2000	1800–2200
	14–18	1800	2000	2400
Male	4–8	1200–1400	1400–1600	1600–2000
	9–13	1600–2000	1800–2200	2000–2600
	14–18	2000–2400	2400–2800	2800–3200

Adapted from US Department of Agriculture, US Department of Health and Human Services. Dietary guidelines for Americans, 2010. 7th edition. Washington, DC: US Government Printing Office; 2010.

overcome by following time-saving, standardized exercise prescription protocols, such as the one developed in Project PACE (see www.paceprojec.org).[17] Evaluation of the PACE program by physicians indicated that 75% would recommend PACE to other physicians and more than 50% reported an increase in their patients' activity levels. Physicians can also refer to the US Department of Health and Human Services exercise guidelines for prescription development. According to these guidelines, children should be advised to perform 60 or more minutes of physical activity each day. This can include either moderate-intensity aerobic activity, such as brisk walking, or vigorous-intensity activity, such as running. Children should also include vigorous-intensity aerobic activity on at least 3 days per week. Muscle strengthening activities, such as gymnastics or push-ups, should be included at least 3 days per week as part of their total 60 or more minutes per day.[18] Other activities, such as swimming, biking, and tennis, are comparable if performed at equivalent intensity and duration. It is important for the physician to remember that weight-loss/maintenance and overall well-being are facilitated by regular exercise.[19]

PHARMACOTHERAPY: NONPRESCRIPTION PRODUCTS

The long-term lifestyle changes necessary to produce and maintain weight loss are difficult. Therefore, nonprescription weight loss products have become prevalent and are attractive to consumers. In fact, the sale of nonprescription weight loss products has turned into a multibillion dollar industry. A recent multistate survey indicated that 7% of respondents (N = 14,679) used a nonprescription weight lose product in the last 2 years.[20] This extrapolates to 17.2 million Americans that have used nonprescription drugs for weight loss.[20] This is a significant health concern, because dietary supplements are regulated as food, not drugs, and are therefore not subject to the same scrutiny as medications. This can result in labeling and dosing inaccuracies that may increase negative health risks.

Ephedrine and phenylpropanolamine (PPA) have been commonly used as appetite suppressants, whereas other products offer meal replacement options (Slimfast, Sweet-Success, and so forth). Because of the potential for adverse effects, ephedrine and PPA are discussed in detail. Ephedrine products have stimulant properties and are purported to decrease weight and appetite.[21,22] In April 2000, restrictions placed on dietary supplements containing ephedrine, in place for 3 years, were withdrawn, citing the need for additional information on adverse effects.[23,24] Adverse effects are currently being studied, but the Food and Drug Administration has recommended labeling that requests those with diabetes, hypertension, and heart disease to seek the advice of a physician before using the products.

PPA is a synthetic ephedrine alkaloid. Until recently, it was thought to be a safe appetite suppressant and stimulant, but case reports of cerebrovascular and cardiac events prompted the voluntary withdrawal of PPA-containing products in November 2000.[25]

In addition, ephedrine and caffeine have been tested for weight loss, but are not approved to treat obesity at this time. Although there are many herbal weight loss products on the market, they are not recommended as a part of a weight management program because these preparations may have unpredictable amounts of active ingredients.

PHARMACOTHERAPY: PRESCRIPTION PRODUCTS

In general, pharmacotherapy for weight reduction achieves about a 10% weight reduction and requires continued compliance to avoid weight gain. Prescription weight loss therapy is based on reducing caloric absorption, decreasing appetite, or increasing metabolic rate. Currently, there is only one prescription weight loss drug available in the United States for adolescents: orilistat (Xenical), approved for adolescents older than 12. According to the Mayo Clinic, prescription medication is not recommended for adolescents because the long-term risks of weight loss medication are still unknown, and it should not be viewed as a replacement for behavioral therapies including healthy diet and exercise. Adolescents should only be treated with orilistat if their BMI is above the level as indicated in **Table 3**.

Orilistat

Orilistat is a pancreatic lipase inhibitor that acts to reduce fatty acid absorption in the intestine. Because the drug is minimally absorbed, it is considered to be generally safe, but is contraindicated in patients with chronic malabsorption syndrome or cholestasis. Its side effects include malabsorption of fat-soluble vitamins and steatorrhea (oily, loose stools with excessive flatus caused by unabsorbed fats reaching the large intestine), and patients taking orilistat should be counseled to take a multivitamin that includes fat-soluble vitamins daily. The usual dosage is 120 mg, three times a day (one per meal) with meals. If a meal is missed or does not contain fat, the dose can be skipped.

Future Directions

New advances in the understanding of the molecular mechanisms of satiety and thermogenesis have opened doors and new opportunities for pharmacotherapy. Potential strategies include targeting leptin, believed to be an afferent signal for satiety in mice. Additionally, melanocortin receptor agonists, cocaine- and amphetamine-regulated transcript receptor agonists, and drugs that target thermogenesis regulation are being studied and may show promise. However, it is unlikely that a "magic pill" that allows weight loss without dietary and activity modification will ever be developed.[25]

BEHAVIOR THERAPY

A National Institutes of Health/National Heart, Lung, and Blood Institute expert panel recommends that behavior therapy be an adjunct treatment of weight loss and weight

Table 3		
BMI guidelines for orilistat (Xenical) treatment		
Age (y)	**BMI Male**	**BMI Female**
12	26.02	26.67
12.5	26.43	27.24
13	26.84	27.76
13.5	27.25	28.20
14	27.63	28.57
14.5	27.98	28.87
15	28.30	29.11
15.5	28.60	29.29
16	28.88	29.43
16.5	29.14	29.56
17	29.41	29.69
17.5	29.70	29.84

maintenance.[9] This treatment modality is important because it assists the patient in identifying cravings and establishing ways to disconnect the triggering events that lead to overeating. Studies show that when behavior therapy is combined with diet therapy in the form of a low-calorie diet or very-low-calorie diet, maintenance of weight loss at 1 year is better than diet alone.[26,27] Studies have shown that behavior therapy increases the effectiveness of pharmacotherapy.[28] It is our recommendation that counseling be part of any weight-reduction program, not only to increase effectiveness, but to help handle the emotional impact that body image can cause.

SUMMARY

Obesity is a significant health problem that is associated with multiple disease states. Family physicians are in a unique role to influence behaviors, such as diet and exercise. When combined with behavior therapy, diet and exercise should be first-line treatment modalities. Pharmacotherapy has been proved effective, but has reluctantly been used by professionals because these drugs have potential side effects, and offer only short-term weight loss. In extreme obese conditions bariatric surgery may be considered after all other less aggressive treatment modalities have failed.

REFERENCES

1. Ogden CL, Carroll MD, Kit BK, et al. Prevalence of childhood and adult obesity in the United States, 2011–2012. JAMA 2014;311(8):806–14.
2. National Center for Health Statistics. Health, United States, 2011: with special features on socioeconomic status and health. Hyattsville (MD): U.S. Department of Health and Human Services; 2012.
3. Serdula MK, Ivery D, Coates RJ, et al. Do obese children become obese adults? A review of the literature. Prev Med 1993;22:167–77.
4. Dietz W. Health consequences of obesity in youth: childhood predictors of adult disease. Pediatrics 1998;101:518–25.
5. Barlow SE, The Expert Committee. Expert committee recommendations regarding the prevention, assessment, and treatment of child and adolescent overweight and obesity: summary report. Pediatrics 2007;120(Suppl):S164–92.
6. Foster GD, Wadden TA, Vogt RA, et al. What is a reasonable weight loss? Patients' expectations and evaluations of obesity treatment outcomes. J Consult Clin Psychol 1997;65(1):79–85.
7. National Institutes of Health, National Heart, Lung, and Blood Institute. Disease and conditions index: what are overweight and obesity? Bethesda (MD): National Institutes of Health; 2010.
8. Fowler-Brown A, Kahwati LC. Prevention and treatment of overweight in children and adolescents. Am Fam Physician 2004;69(11):2591–9.
9. National Institutes of Health, National Heart, Lung, and Blood Institute. North American Association for the Study of Obesity 1998. The practical guide, the identification, evaluation, and treatment of overweight and obesity in adults. Bethesda (MD): NIH. NIH publication no. 00–4084. 1998.
10. Epstein LH, Goldfield GS. Physical activity in the treatment of childhood overweight and obesity: current evidence and research issues. Med Sci Sports Exerc 1999;31(11 Suppl):S553–9.
11. U.S. Department of Agriculture, U.S. Department of Health and Human Services. Dietary guidelines for Americans, 2010. 7th edition. Washington, DC: US Government Printing Office; 2010.

12. Pate RR, Pratt M, Blair SN, et al. Physical activity and public health: a recommendation from the Centers for Disease Control and Prevention and the American College of Sports Medicine. JAMA 1995;273:402–7.

13. Foreyt JP, Goodrick GK. Attributes of successful approaches to weight loss and control. Appl Prev Psychol 1994;3:209–15.

14. US Preventive Task Force. Guide to clinical preventive services. 2nd edition. Baltimore (MD): Williams & Wilkins; 1996.

15. Logsdon DN, Lazaro CM, Meier RV. The feasibility of behavioral risk reduction in primary medical care. Am J Prev Med 1989;5:249–56.

16. Wee CC, McCarthy EP, Davis RB, et al. Physician counseling about exercise. JAMA 1999;282(16):1583–8.

17. Patrick K, Sallis JF, Long BJ, et al. A new tool for encouraging activity: project PACE. The Physician and Sportsmedicine 1994;22(11):45–55.

18. U.S. Department of Health and Human Services. Physical activity guidelines for Americans Midcourse Report Subcommittee of the President's Council on Fitness, Sports & Nutrition. Physical activity guidelines for Americans Midcourse Report: strategies to increase physical activity among youth. Washington, DC: U.S. Department of Health and Human Services; 2012.

19. Kayman S, Bruvold W, Stern JS. Maintenance and relapse after weight loss in women: behavioral aspects. Am J Clin Nutr 1990;52:800–7.

20. Blank HM, Kahn LK, Serdula MK. Use of nonprescription weight loss products: results from a multistate survey. JAMA 2001;266(8):930–5.

21. Astrup A, Toubro S, Cannon S, et al. Thermogenic synergism between ephedrine and caffeine in healthy volunteers: a double-blind, placebo-controlled study. Metabolism 1991;40:323–9.

22. Allison DB, Fontaine KR, Heshika S, et al. Alternative treatments for weight loss: a critical review. Crit Rev Food Sci Nutr 2001;41:1–28.

23. Food and Drug Administration. Dietary supplements containing ephedrine alkalosis. 62 Federal Register 30677-37024. Silver Spring (MD): Food and Drug Administration, Department of Health and Human Services. 1997.

24. Food and Drug Administration. Public health advisory subject: safety of phenylpropanamine. Silver Spring (MD): Food and Drug Administration, Department of Health and Human Services. 2000.

25. Mun ED, Blackburn GL, Matthews JB. Current status of medical and surgical therapy for obesity. Gastroenterology 2001;120:669–81.

26. Wadden TA, Stunkard AJ. Controlled trial of very low calorie diet, behavior therapy, and their combination in the treatment of obesity. J Consult Clin Psychol 1986;54:482–8.

27. Wadden TA, Stunkard AJ. One-year behavioral treatment of obesity: comparison of moderate and severe caloric restriction and the effects of weight maintenance therapy. J Consult Clin Psychol 1994;62:165–71.

28. Knutson D, Craighead LW, Stunkard AJ, et al. Behavior therapy and pharmacotherapy for obesity. Arch Gen Psychiatry 1981;38:763–8.

Printed and bound by CPI Group (UK) Ltd, Croydon, CR0 4YY

03/10/2024

01040489-0015